# Infertility

*by the same author*

The Menopause

Pregnancy After Thirty

An A–Z of Gynaecology

A Handbook of Obstetrics and Gynaecology
for the House Officer

The Anatomy and Physiology
of Obstetrics (reviser)

# Infertility

## A guide for the anxious couple

Mary Anderson
MB, ChB, FRCOG

ff
*faber and faber*
LONDON · BOSTON

First published in 1987
by Faber and Faber Limited
3 Queen Square London WC1N 3AU

Photoset and printed in Great Britain by
Redwood Burn Limited, Trowbridge, Wiltshire


*British Library Cataloguing in Publication Data*

Anderson, Mary
Infertility : a guide for the anxious couple.
1. Infertility—Treatment
I. Title
616.6'9206 RC889

ISBN 0–571–13856–X

# Contents

# Illustrations



**Tables**

# Acknowledgements

My thanks are due to Miss P. Downie, Medical and Nursing Editor, Faber and Faber, for not only suggesting the idea of this book but also for her ever ready encouragement and support.

I must also thank Mrs K. Maclean who, in spite of heavy commitments, typed the manuscript speedily and with precision.

Figure 5/3 is reproduced from *Fundamentals of Obstetrics and Gynaecology*, volume 2 Gynaecology, 4th edition, by Derek Llewellyn-Jones. It it included by permission of the publishers, Faber and Faber, London.

# Introduction

Almost always the desired outcome of a happy marriage or stable relationship is children. The natural expectation of any healthy young couple is that when they plan a pregnancy it will be achieved without undue delay. Unfortunately this is by no means always so and nothing seems to engender greater anxiety than failure to conceive. This anxiety in itself may not only cause further delay in conception but introduce such strain into a relationship as may be intolerable.

Understanding of a problem goes half-way to solving it and this is true of conception and delay in conception. Reading this book will not, of course, magic away basic clinical problems but, hopefully, if such exist an understanding of them will at least lessen anxiety and create an attitude of patience with investigations and investigators alike and always an attitude of optimism.

# 1

# The Problem of Infertility

Failure to conceive affects 10 to 15 per cent of all couples. Far from being a gloomy opening comment to this book, these figures should mean that an infertile couple need not feel isolated with their problem. This may give some encouragement if not comfort and, in fact, meeting other couples in an infertility clinic and perhaps sharing experiences may be quite an important aspect of management. Others will want to be alone with their problem, pursuing investigations in privacy, and this attitude must always be respected. One of the difficulties, of course, is the pressure of well-intentioned relatives who not only press for information but, what is worse, give unasked for – and more often than not, false – advice. Every effort has to be made both to ignore these gratuitous remarks but certainly also to check them with the investigating doctor if they give rise to a persistent worry.

Although, as one authority has put it, in most women 'the desire for children is stronger than self-interest in beauty and figure, stronger than the claims of a career' nevertheless in present times pregnancy may be delayed until older ages – late twenties early thirties. Perhaps this in itself accounts for a larger proportion of couples who are 'relatively infertile' – that is, where there is a delay in conception. This is not to imply that earlier conception should be preferred. By no means. These things are ordered by personal choice and social custom in most instances. But what it does mean is that the older couple should not be too surprised if pregnancy does not instantly occur when planned. If, as time elapses, they have to embark on a series of investigations they should be patient, knowing that it may take a little longer for them before success is achieved.

## When is infertility diagnosed?

Investigations are usually begun when a couple have been trying to conceive for a year – with normal frequency of intercourse taking place during this time. 'Normal frequency' is usually taken to mean two or three times each week and although full orgasm on the part of the woman is not essential full penetration must be achieved and there should not be significant deep pain felt by the woman, which may be indicative of pelvic disease.

This one-year 'rule' is made to be broken of course – investigations may be started earlier in the case of an older couple, especially if coital difficulties exist, or later in young people, who may be just a little too enthusiastic to seek help.

It may give some reassurance to know these approximate facts:

70 per cent of couples have conceived after 1 year
80 per cent after 18 months
90 per cent after 2 years.

## What are the investigations?

These will be discussed in detail in later chapters but let us note certain points. First, it takes two to make a baby, so the gynaecologist will want to interview both man and woman and investigations will be arranged for both. Although the attitude is becoming much less common, some men cannot accept the possibility that they may have a problem and so refuse investigation.

There are ways of overcoming this as we shall see and the

writer feels that no criticism should be levelled at the man by the doctor, especially to the woman. This can only increase tension, which is hardly the background for successful conception. The couple should be encouraged to talk things over and it is surprising how often this is successful in achieving mutual co-operation.

In outline, investigations for the male partner will be on his semen, and for the female partner on her ovaries and whether they are producing eggs satisfactorily, on her tubes and whether they are functioning normally, on her uterus and cervix and their capabilities, and of course on the ability of her partner's sperm to enter her genital tract and reach an egg successfully. These points will all be discussed in greater detail in later chapters.

One very important point to remember. Ovulation (the production of an egg) takes place, at best, only once a month. This fact alone means that investigations will take time. It cannot just be a question of an initial consultation then one or two tests, the results of which are obtained in a few days, some advice or treatment and then – hey, presto! Careful, painstaking search has to be made and weeks inevitably pass. But if they lead to success then time does not matter.

## Who are the investigators?

Usually a couple worried about their failure to conceive will first seek advice from their own family doctor. And this is how it should be. To talk to someone whom you know and who knows you is so important if only for the fact that you feel more relaxed, so when you do embark on investigations with a specialist you will be backed up by the understanding and confidence which your own doctor has already given you.

After your doctor's preliminary questions and examination – and he may arrange for some initial laboratory investigations – you will be referred to a hospital for further assessment. Depending on your local facilities, this will be either to a gynaecological clinic or to an infertility clinic. Some hospitals are able to provide special clinics for this work staffed by doctors whose particular interest is in the management of infertile couples. Some individuals will seek the help of a private gynaecologist. It is important, however, always to consult your own doctor first for he is likely to know the best person to whom to refer you for this particular problem.

The people you are likely to meet during your investigations are:

1. *The gynaecologist*: This specialist in the problems of women is well versed in the problem of infertility and will talk to you at some length, examine you and initiate the investigations which we shall discuss later. It is at this initial interview that it is so important that both partners should attend if possible. Incidentally, you may meet the gynaecologist's registrar, his assistant. Do not be disappointed. These young men, or women, are specialists in training and will be well versed in the problem of infertility.

2. *The urologist*: If the male has to be examined or investigated further it is customary to refer him to a 'male specialist'. This is the urologist. Rarely does a gynaecologist examine the male partner physically – this is done by the urologist.

3. *The radiologist*: This is the *x*-ray specialist and, nowadays, the specialist in ultrasound scanning. Depending on the findings of the gynaecologist's examination, further *x*-ray tests or examination by scanning may be arranged. These will be discussed later.

4. *The laboratory*: As you will see later, laboratory tests are an essential part of infertility investigations. The woman will have a sample of blood taken; her partner will have his

semen examined in the laboratory and possibly the urologist will arrange for a blood test later, if required.

These then are the initial comments on this problem of delay in conceiving. Let us now tackle the problem step by step. First we must examine what is required to achieve a pregnancy – the organs involved and their function. Then we must consider how we test the function of each of these prerequisites. Finally, we shall see how problems can be identified and what methods can be employed in treating them.

# 2

# Anatomy and Physiology

A basic knowledge of the anatomical structures and the way in which they function in order to achieve a pregnancy is essential. This will provide a better understanding of what is happening – and, of course, what may not be happening – and an appreciation of the time factor that must inevitably be involved in the investigation of the infertile couple. If the readers complete this chapter and then think back on what they have read it will perhaps be true to say that they may well find it surprising that so many people *do* achieve pregnancy without apparent difficulty. The events leading to conception are complex and in many ways haphazard. Chance plays quite a large part as we shall see.

**The anatomy of the male reproductive organs** (Fig. 2/1)

The male sex organs consist of the *penis* and two *testes* (testicles) which are enclosed in the pouch called the *scrotum*. The scrotum is covered by thin pigmented ridged skin and underneath the skin is a layer of muscle called the dartos muscle. The scrotum is divided into two compartments in which lie the testes, the left one at a lower level than the right.

The testes are the source of sperm cells and the male hormone testosterone. Each testis is composed of multiple lobules, each one containing the seminiferous tubules which are coiled structures closely packed within each lobule. Each lobule communicates behind with small channels which empty into larger ducts and these pierce the covering capsule

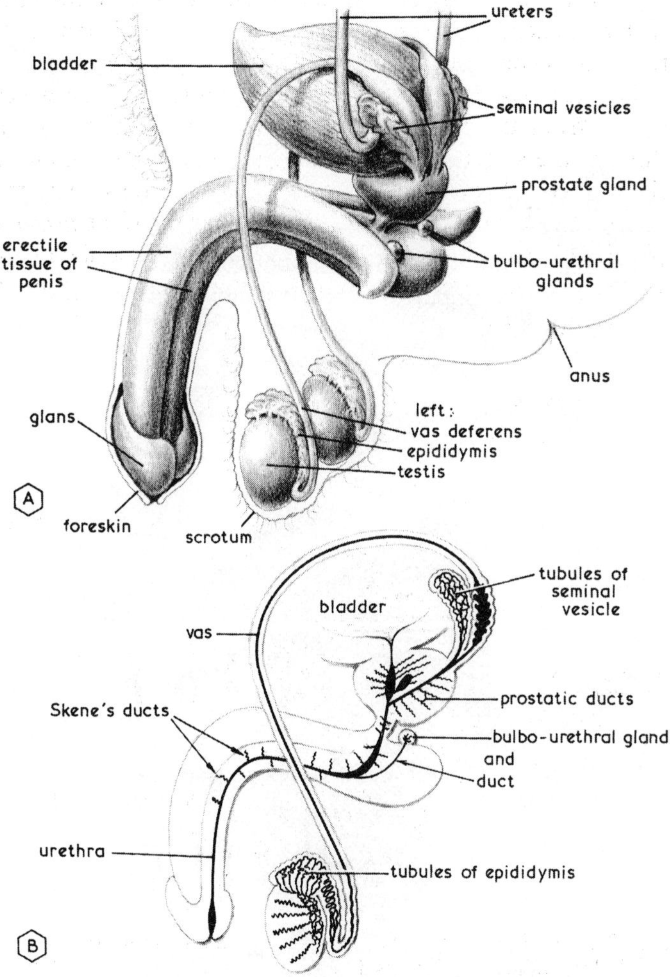


Fig. 2/1 The male reproductive organs

of the testis at its upper part to pass into a structure called the *epididymis*. These ducts, called efferent ducts, fuse together within the head of the epididymis to form a convoluted single tube which constitutes the body and tail of the epididymis.

The *vas deferens* is a tube about 45cm (18in) long which passes from the tail of the epididymis up into the pelvis through the scrotum to join the penis. The penis contains a channel called the *urethra* and the vas deferens joins the urethra by passing through *ejaculatory ducts* and the *prostate gland*. This gland is a small pyramidal shaped glandular organ surrounding the upper urethra. It contributes secretions to the seminal fluid.

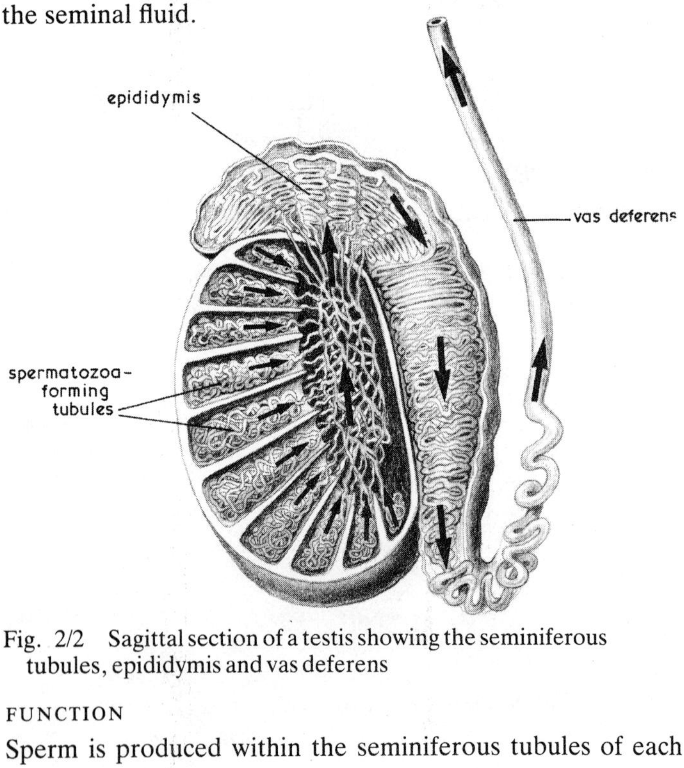


Fig. 2/2 Sagittal section of a testis showing the seminiferous tubules, epididymis and vas deferens

FUNCTION

Sperm is produced within the seminiferous tubules of each

testis by a process known as *spermatogenesis* (Fig. 2/2). The sperm enters the network of tubules and finally reaches the epididymis. There further development of the sperm cells takes place and they are moved along by muscular contractions of the tube known as peristalsis. The sperm then enters the vas deferens and travels up to the prostate. Where the vas deferens meets the urethra there is a small sac-like structure called the seminal vesicle and here the sperm is stored. From the seminal vesicles the sperm, bathed in secretions largely from the prostate, pass into the urethra and are released from the tip of the penis (the *glans*).

### SEXUAL INTERCOURSE

When sexual intercourse takes place the erect penis is inserted into the female vagina and as a result of friction between the sensitive tip (glans) of the penis and the vaginal wall, seminal fluid is ejected into the vagina.

Erection of the penis is brought about by the distension of the venous sinuses in the substance of the penis altering the normally flaccid organ into a rigid elongated structure which will allow the semen to be deposited high up in the vagina near the entrance to the uterus.

Reflex action during the act of intercourse closes the entrance to the bladder so that the seminal fluid cannot enter the bladder (nor is urine passed) but is propelled along the channels to be discharged from the urethra. Emission of semen is associated in the male with the peak of sexual excitement which is called *orgasm*.

### SPERMATOZOA

We have seen that spermatozoa are formed from cells in the seminiferous tubules of the testes. They undergo several changes before becoming mature and one vital change is the reduction by half of the chromosome complement of each spermatozoon.

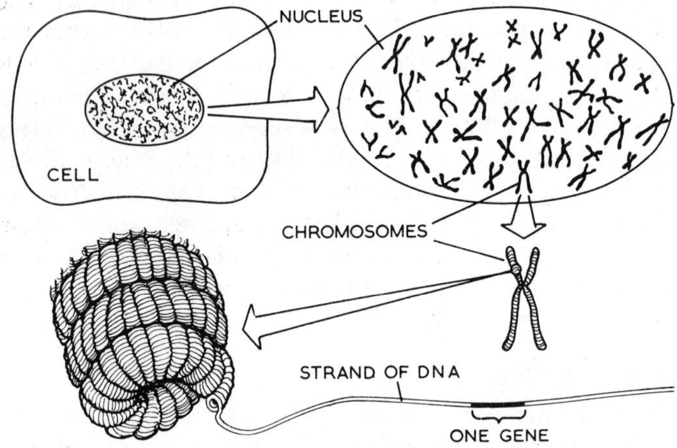


Fig. 2/3 Make-up of a cell

In the centre of every cell in the body is the nucleus and within the nucleus are twisted strands of material called chromosomes. These chromosomes play a fundamental part in the transmission of hereditary characteristics. Strung along the length of the chromosomes like beads, are the genes. These consist of a substance called deoxyribonucleic acid (DNA) and they are responsible for 'handing on' the properties of the parent cell (Fig. 2/3).

Now every cell in the human body – apart from the spermatozoa in the male and the ova (or egg cells) in the female – contains 46 chromosomes: 44 are concerned with physical characteristics and are called autosomes, the other two determine the sex of the individual.

The mature spermatozoon, like the mature ovum, has 23 chromosomes (22 autosomes and 1 sex chromosome). When the mature sperm fuses with the ovum, therefore, the total complement of 44 autosomes and 2 sex chromosomes is reached. Both sex chromosomes in the female are identical, have the shape of an X and are called the X chromosomes. In the male the two sex chromosomes are different, the smallest one looking like a Y so the male cell complement is XY.

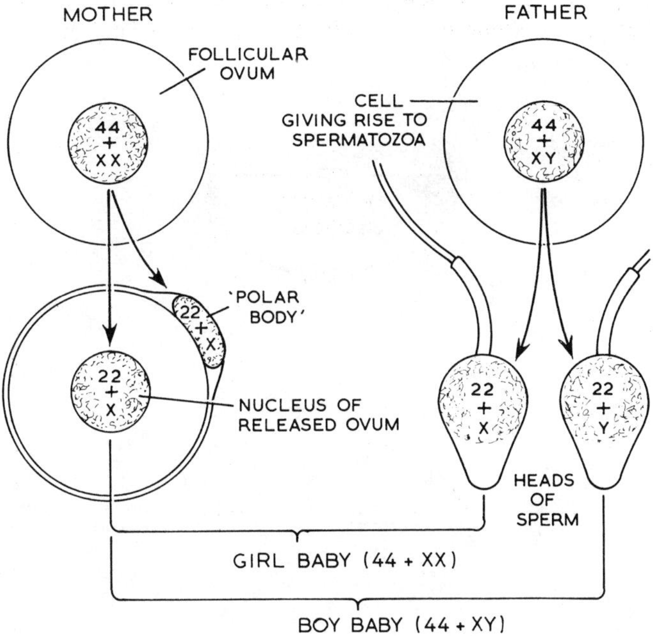


Fig. 2/4 Determining the baby's sex

When the maturing spermatozoon divides to have half its complement of chromosomes the two sex chromosomes contribute either an X or a Y chromosome to the 22 autosomes of each spermatozoon. Obviously when fusion with an ovum takes place the sex chromosomes will either be XX (a girl) or XY ( boy) (Fig. 2/4).

In this way the father is the partner who determines the sex of the baby.

*Structure of a spermatozoon*

The appearance of a spermatozoon (sperm for convenience) is shown in Figure 2/5. It consists of a head, which contains the chromosomes, a middle piece concerned with supplying energy, and a tail which propels it through the female genital tract. Its total length is about 0.05mm and it can be seen only under the microscope.

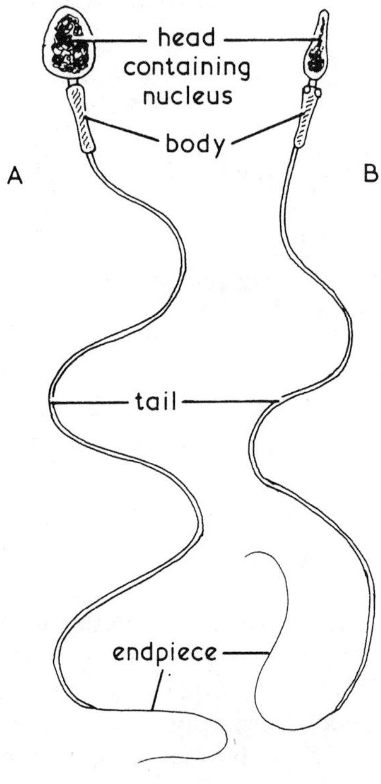


Fig. 2/5 A spermatozoon. A. Showing the various parts. B. Side view

Unlike the female who is born with her full complement of egg cells only one of which is shed at ovulation once a month, the male continuously produces spermatozoa and millions are deposited in the vagina at each intercourse. As we shall see later the journey for the sperms thereafter is hazardous, only a few thousands passing through the cervix into the uterine cavity, only a few hundred entering the tube and only a dozen or so passing along the tube with one finally penetrating the covering of the egg cell.

*Hormone control of sperm production*

A hormone called follicle stimulating hormone (FSH), from the pituitary gland, probably initiates spermatogenesis from the testicular tubes.

Also from the pituitary gland a second hormone called luteinising hormone (LH) stimulates specialised testicular cells to produce testosterone. This hormone facilitates spermatogenesis as well as stimulating the apparatus which we have seen transports the sperm.

It takes 60 to 65 days to complete the production of sperm and then another 10 to 12 days for their journey through the epididymis and vas deferens to the seminal vesicles where they are to be stored pending ejaculation.

Now let us take a look at the female anatomy concerned with reproduction.

**The anatomy of the female reproductive organs**

The female sex organs consist of the external genitalia, the *vulva*, and the internal genitalia which are the *vagina*, the *uterus*, the *tubes* and the *ovaries*.

THE VULVA (Fig. 2/6)

This consists of several structures surrounding the entrance to the vagina.

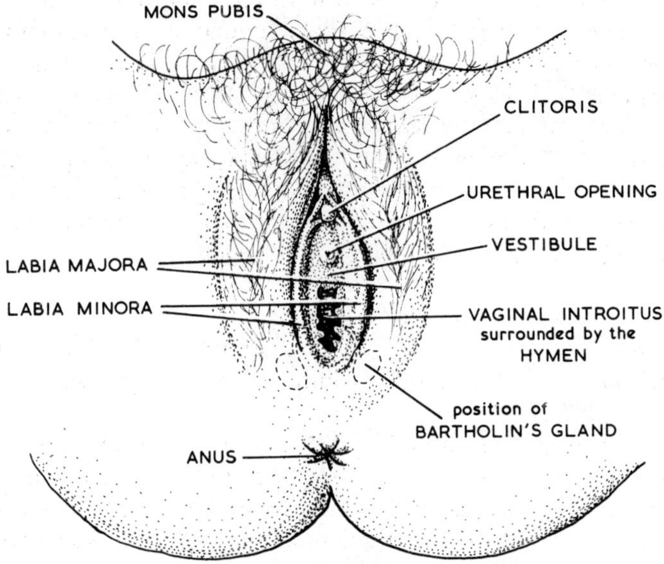


Fig. 2/6 The female external genitalia

1. *The labia majora* or 'large lips', are two large folds of skin filled with fat and containing hair follicles and sweat glands. In front, they merge into a pad of fat, the *mons pubis*, lying over the pubic bone and covered by skin and hairs. Behind, the labia are thinner and merge into the wedge of muscular tissue lying between the back border of the *vagina* and the opening of the bowel (the *anus*). This wedge is called the *perineal body*.

2. *The labia minora* or 'small lips', are two folds of pink skin lying inside the labia majora and immediately on either side of the entrance or 'vestibule' of the vagina. They contain no hair and little fat but many blood vessels.

3. *The clitoris* is the female equivalent of the male penis and is about 2.5cm long. It consists of erectile tissue which becomes engorged with blood during sexual excitement and can lead to orgasm if directly stimulated. The front part of the labia majora splits into two folds to surround it.

4. *The hymen* is a thin incomplete membrane which surrounds the opening to the vagina (the *introitus*). After sexual intercourse has begun, or after the use of tampons, only tags of the hymen remain. These are called the *carunculae myrtiformes*.

On either side of the introitus, outside the hymen, are two collections of erectile tissue which also fill with blood during sexual excitement. They are the *vestibular bulbs*. At their lower ends are two small glands with ducts opening on the surface just inside the lower end of the labia minora. These are the *Bartholin's glands* which secrete mucus to provide lubrication during sexual intercourse.

THE INTERNAL GENITALIA (Fig. 2/7)

These lie inside the body and are closely concerned with reproduction – indeed they are the organs of reproduction.

*The vagina*

This is a hollow muscular tube about 9cm long leading from the vulva below to the uterus above. The front and back walls lie in apposition but as the walls are lined by skin containing multiple folds the vagina is capable of considerable stretching such as occurs during sexual intercourse and particularly during childbirth. At the upper end of the vagina is the neck of the uterus – *the cervix* – projecting through the vault of the vagina.

*The uterus and cervix*

The uterus (womb) is a hollow pear-shaped organ lying above the vagina within the pelvis. It measures approximately

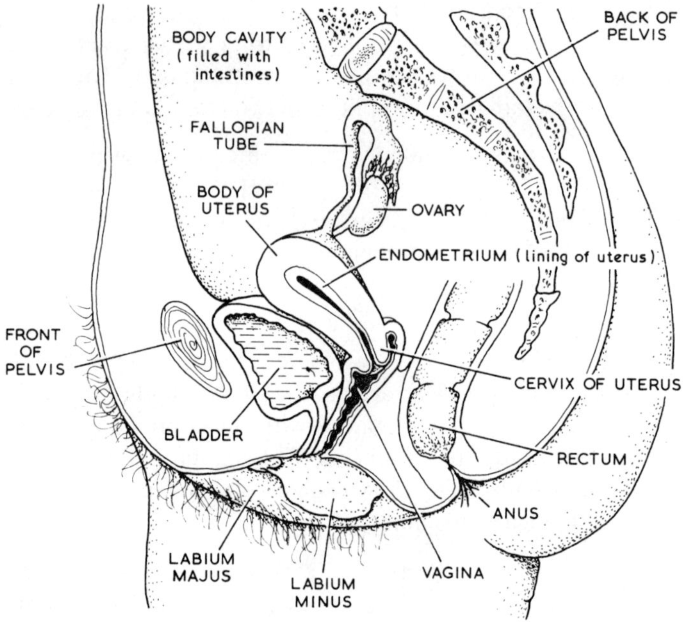


Fig. 2/7 The female reproductive organs

7.6cm in length, 5cm in width at its widest part, and weighs about 60g. Its muscular walls are about 1.5cm thick and its cavity, normally just a slit, is capable of enormous distension which, of course, happens during the growth of a pregnancy.

The main part of the uterus lying above the vagina is called the *body* and the narrower portion projecting into the vagina, the *neck* (*cervix*).

Lining the cavity of the body of the uterus is specialised tissue called *endometrium*. This grows thick during a menstrual cycle and, if a pregnancy does not occur, is shed during menstruation.

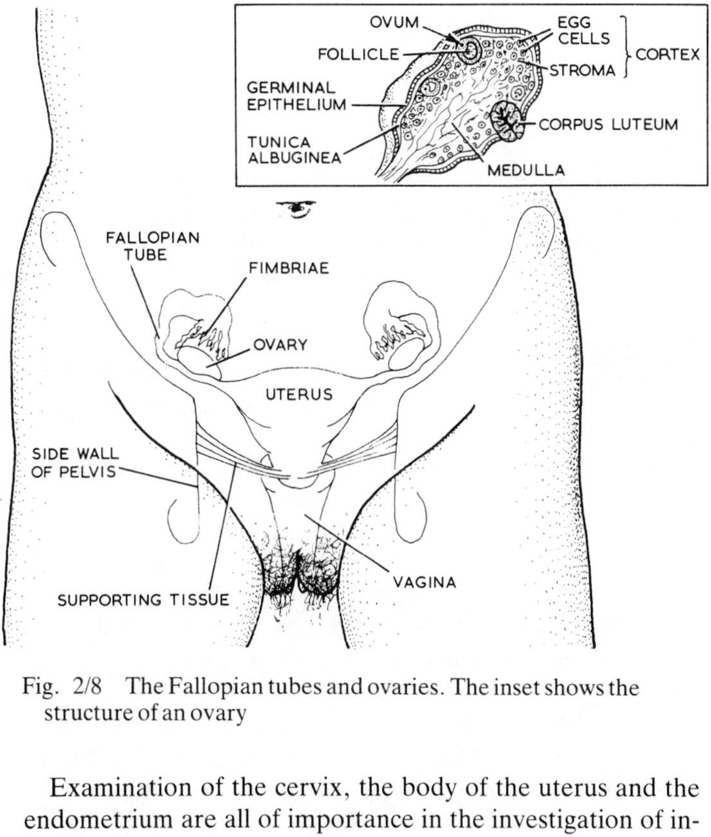


Fig. 2/8 The Fallopian tubes and ovaries. The inset shows the structure of an ovary

Examination of the cervix, the body of the uterus and the endometrium are all of importance in the investigation of infertility.

*The tubes and ovaries* (Fig. 2/8)

The *tubes* (Fallopian tubes is the full anatomical title) are two hollow tube-like structures about 10cm long which project out from either side of the upper part of the body of the uterus. At their outer ends they hang over the ovaries with finger-like processes called *fimbriae* providing a connecting link between the ovaries and the cavity of the uterus. The fimbriae are so constructed that they 'pick up' an egg from the surface of the ovary. The egg is then carried along the tube, helped partly by the muscular activity of the walls of the tube and partly by the special cells lining the tube. These possess hair-like processes which waft the egg along. Fertilisation of the egg takes place within the tube and the fertilised egg is then carried to the cavity of the uterus where it implants in the thickened lining now known as the *decidua*.

From this description it is obvious that a study of the tubes – their patency and their function – will be an essential part of investigations into problems of infertility.

With the ovaries we come to one of the central requirements for reproduction. Here it is that the eggs or ova are produced.

The *ovaries* are two almond-shaped bodies, whitish in colour and corrugated in appearance. They are approximately 3cm long, 2cm broad and weigh about 6g. The outer coat is called the *cortex* and is the functioning part of the ovary containing the egg cells embedded in a layer of cells called the *stroma*. In the centre of each ovary is the part known as the *medulla* which contains its blood vessels and nerves.

The ovaries are, in a sense, the equivalent of the male testes. At the onset of maturity, however, they contain the entire quota of egg cells – about 200 000 – and only one will mature with each menstrual cycle. This is different from the male where we have seen that sperm are produced by a continuous manufacturing process.

The ovaries also secrete the female hormones which are an integral part of the production of eggs – *ovulation* – and either menstruation or conception.

#### FUNCTION

The cyclical functioning of the female reproductive organs is a complicated series of events, but for our purpose in seeing where problems arise in achieving a pregnancy it can be simplified.

In the mature female when a pregnancy is not achieved, regular menstruation will take place. The control of menstruation is shown in Figure 2/9 and, summarised, the events are as follows:

1. A portion of the brain called the hypothalamus produces hormones which affect the front part of the pituitary gland – a pea-sized structure lying at the base of the brain. (Incidentally a hormone is a chemical substance produced by a gland and carried in the bloodstream to affect and act on different parts of the body.) These hormones from the hypothalamus are termed releasing hormones and the hormones they release from the pituitary gland are:

The follicle – stimulating hormone (FSH)
The luteinising hormone (LH).

2. Mainly FSH is produced in the first part of a monthly cycle and has the effect of stimulating the 'follicles' in the ovary which contains the egg cells or ova. These follicles ripen and several come to the surface of the ovary. One of these ripe follicles reaches the surface of the ovary first and ruptures, releasing the egg or ovum. Ovulation has taken place.

3. This event of ovulation is initiated by a surge of luteinising hormone (LH). The reason for this surge is as follows: the ripening follicles produce the hormone oestrogen and oestrogen has a 'negative' effect on the pituitary, reducing the production of FSH. As the levels of oestrogen in the blood continue to rise it then has a 'positive' effect on the pituitary producing a sudden marked rise in LH at about mid-cycle. It is this surge in LH which induces ovulation.

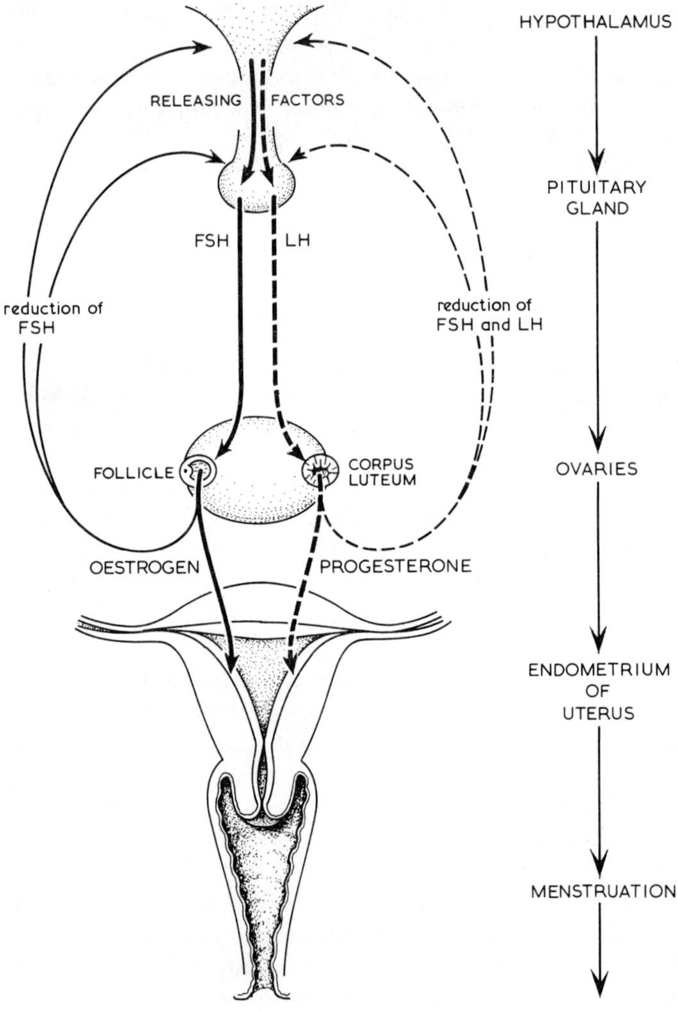


Fig. 2/9 The control of menstruation

4. After ovulation has taken place the empty follicle collapses to form a tiny yellowish-red structure on the surface of the ovary. This is called the *corpus luteum* and from this structure comes the second main female hormone called progesterone. Together with oestrogen, progesterone acts on the hypothalamus and pituitary in a negative way and the levels of FSH and LH fall.

5. Meantime the endometrium (the specialised lining of the cavity of the uterus) undergoes significant changes. These are designed to prepare for the reception and 'bedding down' of a fertilised ovum if fertilisation should occur in that cycle.

During the first half of the cycle the endometrium is stimulated by the rising levels of oestrogen and, having repaired itself following the preceding menstruation, it becomes thick and vascular. This is called the *proliferative* phase.

During the second half of the cycle the effect of progesterone is seen on the endometrium. It gets much thicker, is full of glands filled with secretion and develops a rich blood supply. This is the *secretory* phase of the endometrium and provides a suitable nourishing 'bed' in which a fertilised egg can settle and begin to grow.

If fertilisation has not occurred then the levels of oestrogen and progesterone drop, the thick endometrium can no longer be supported and it sheds itself from the uterus as the menstrual flow.

This sequence of events is quite complicated to understand and Figure 2/10 and Table 2/1 may help to clarify menstrual physiology.

The timing of the various events is variable but it is important to remember that ovulation – the production of the egg – tends to occur 14 days before the *next* menstrual period. In a 28-day cycle this is, of course, mid-cycle but many women have longer or shorter cycles (e.g. in a 35-day cycle ovulation

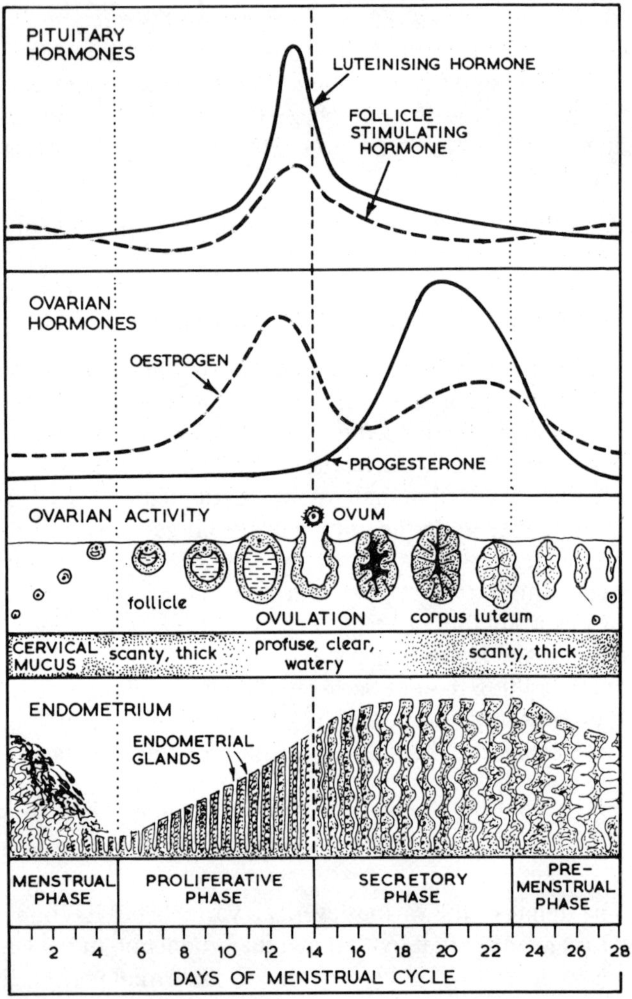


Fig. 2/10 A sequence explaining the physiology of menstruation and ovulation

would occur on or about day 21) and it is important for them to remember this 'ovulation rule' when they are trying to become pregnant.

**Table 2/1** The events leading to menstruation

| | | *No. of days* |
|---|---|---|
| 1. | After menstruation a follicle ripens: oestrogen is produced: the endometrium proliferates | 10 |
| 2. | Ovulation | |
| 3. | The corpus luteum appears: progesterone is produced: small amounts of oestrogen persist: the endometrium becomes secretory | 14 |
| 4. | The corpus luteum degenerates: oestrogen and progesterone levels fall: menstruation | 4 |
| | TOTAL | 28 |

**The mechanism of conception** (Fig. 2/11)

We have seen that millions of sperm are deposited in the upper vagina when the man ejaculates during intercourse. Ejaculation occurs at orgasm in the man but orgasm in the woman is not essential for conception. This is not always realised and can sometimes lead to growing anxiety – which in itself leads to less enjoyment of love making and ultimately decreasing frequency. This vicious cycle is not exactly conducive to conception.

So, what are the events that lead to sperm meeting ovum and resulting in fertilisation?

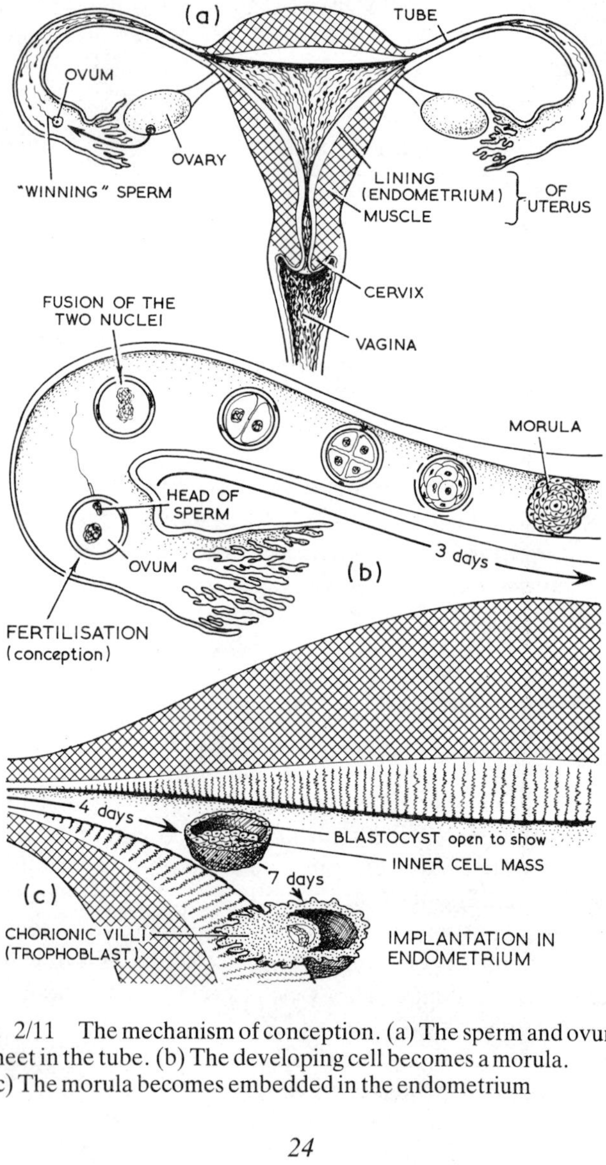


Fig. 2/11 The mechanism of conception. (a) The sperm and ovum meet in the tube. (b) The developing cell becomes a morula. (c) The morula becomes embedded in the endometrium

1. The end of a healthy tube hanging over the ovary has the finger-like processes or fimbriae which we have described. These pick up the ovum or egg as it is shed from the follicle and the ovum thus enters the tube. Here it is moved down towards the uterus by a combination of muscular activity in the tube and the hair-like processes on the surface of the tube's lining cells which waft the egg downwards.

The egg has a life of about 24 to 36 hours.

2. Meanwhile, of the millions of sperm deposited in the upper vagina, many fewer actually reach the cavity of the uterus and only a few hundred ultimately reach the outer portion of the tube where a few will finally meet the ovum (Fig. 2/11a). A few penetrate the outer covering of the ovum but only one gets to the very centre of the ovum fusing with the female nucleus. And then conception has occurred.

Sperm have a life of about 48 hours so for fertilisation to take place intercourse must occur within two days of ovulation.

3. When the ovum is fertilised it divides into a little ball of cells called a *morula* (Fig. 2/11b). The morula is wafted down the tube and reaches the cavity of the uterus about seven days after ovulation which is about day 21 of a 28-day cycle. It settles into the now thickened endometrium and is fully embedded by the 14th day after ovulation, that is about day 28 of the cycle (Fig. 2/11c).

4. We have already seen how the lining of the uterus, the endometrium, becomes thick and lush with plenty of blood supply, in the second half of the cycle. It is this ideal 'nest' which the egg meets when it reaches the cavity of the uterus and there it settles down and begins to grow. The endometrium then becomes known as the decidua and its development is brought about by the continuing influence of the

corpus luteum which, in turn, is directed by the pituitary hormones.

5. To complete the picture the fertilised egg has been changing meantime. By the time the little ball of cells, the morula, has reached the cavity of the uterus a small fluid-filled space has appeared within it to separate it into an outer shell with a mound of cells lying to one side. The outer shell will become the placenta and the mound of cells (the inner cell mass) will be the site of the development of the fetus.

The placenta takes over the production of the hormones required to maintain the corpus luteum which in turn, as we have seen, is producing hormones to sustain the decidua in which the fertilised egg is embedded. Later in pregnancy – after 10 to 12 weeks – the level of these hormones declines, the corpus luteum fails, but the developing placenta takes over the production of oestrogen and progesterone.

Armed with these anatomical and physical facts we can, I think, begin to work out where things can go wrong in attempting to achieve a pregnancy. If we can understand where things go wrong then, generally, it is a short step to understanding how they can be put right. The following chapters will attempt logically, step by step, to examine the 'faults' in the system and then show how these faults can be rectified.

# 3

# What can go Wrong?

First, a definition: infertility means failure to conceive after 12 months of unprotected intercourse. It may be *primary*, which means that there has never been a pregnancy, or *secondary* where there has been a previous pregnancy (whether it reached full time or ended as a miscarriage).

We have already seen that 10 to 15 per cent of couples in the reproductive age group are infertile. The source of the problem may be the woman (approximately 30 per cent) or the man (approximately 30 per cent) or both (approximately 30 per cent). In the remaining 10 per cent no cause can be identified.

Let us look at the possible problems of the male partner and by referring to the description in the previous chapter of his anatomy and its functioning we shall be able to see where faults may arise. In later chapters we shall see how far these faults can be investigated and treated. (It is perhaps wrong to use the word 'fault' in reference to either partner of an infertile couple. 'Fault' has the implication of blame and better words would be 'defect' or 'imperfection' or just 'problem'.)

Fundamentally, infertility of the male will be shown when a microscopic examination of his semen – referred to as semen analysis – reveals inadequate sperm. What constitutes a normal semen analysis? The specimen of semen is collected by masturbation after two or three days of abstaining from intercourse. The specimen is brought in a specially provided plastic container as soon as possible to the laboratory. The figures normally quoted for a normal 'sperm count' or semen analysis are as follows.

| | | |
|---|---|---|
| Volume of sample | | 1–4ml |
| Number of sperm | > | 20–40 million/ml |
| Abnormal forms | < | 20% |
| Motility | | 50–70% |

It is not so much the number of sperm present in the sample that counts but their activity and their normal configuration. More attention to these aspects has been paid in recent years rather than to the actual count. If a first semen count is abnormal then a second must be carried out later. The difficulties which some men experience in trying to produce such a specimen may well be reflected in the count.

### The male factor in infertility

Having established an abnormal count what can be wrong?

1. ABNORMAL ANATOMY

*Hypospadias* is a condition in which the opening of the penis is on the underside possibly some distance back from the tip. Deposition of semen well within the vagina is obviously difficult in such a situation and fertility reduced.

*Cryptorchidism* is a condition in which the testes have remained within the abdomen instead of descending into the scrotum. This is a situation usually diagnosed in earlier life but during the course of examining the male partner of an infertile couple the scrotum will be felt for the presence of both testes.

*Klinefelter's syndrome* is a genetic anomaly in which the chromosomal numbers are abnormal, namely 47 (instead of 46) XXY (instead of XY, the normal male complement). Klinefelter individuals are tall, eunuchoid, with little facial or body hair and have very small inactive testes. Sexual potency is likely but no sperm are present.

*Absence of the vas deferens and/or epididymis*: In this structural abnormality, the route for the sperm from testes to penis is blocked. Vasectomy – the operation for male sterilisation – will do this, of course, but the defect may be the result of a developmental abnormality.

*Varicocele*: This is one of the more common structural defects. It consists of enlarged veins (varicose veins) around the epididymis and vas deferens. Although why this defect should depress the production of sperm is not entirely clear it is thought that the varicosities create a higher local temperature thereby lowering production.

These are the commoner structural defects.

## 2. FUNCTIONAL DEFECTS

### *Hypothalamic-pituitary disorders*

Just as ovulation is controlled by the higher centres of the brain (hypothalamus) through the pituitary gland so is testicular function although there is no cyclical activity as in the female.

FSH and LH are involved as is the hormone testosterone. Deficiency of one or all of these may produce abnormalities of sperm production.

Abnormal function of other glands such as the thyroid or adrenal gland may indirectly affect testicular function.

### *Disorders of the testes*

The production of sperm can be arrested at any stage in the seminiferous tubules. One rare developmental cause is the absence of spermatocytes – the cells which produce the sperm. There is, of course, no method of correcting this fundamental defect.

### *Infection*

Probably the best known infection causing impairment of

spermatogenesis – the production of sperm – is *mumps*. *Orchitis* is an inflammation of the testis causing swelling and pain and may be associated with infection by the mumps virus. When this happens (and it may occur in 25 per cent of men developing mumps) the sperm-producing elements in the testes may be damaged to a greater or lesser extent.

Other infections may cause similar damage – gonococcal, syphilitic and non-specific bacterial infections.

Once damage has occurred as a result of any of these infections it is irreversible.

*Drugs*

Some drugs may affect spermatogenesis. For example, alcohol, tranquillisers and narcotics all depress the production of sperm.

Anti-cancer chemotherapy usually causes *azoospermia* (absence of sperm) and recovery, after therapy is discontinued, is very variable. Obviously anti-cancer therapy when it is needed is a 'must' and in such cases 'banking' of the sperm before the start of therapy may provide an answer.

*Miscellaneous*

Environment plays a part in the normal production of sperm. *Temperature* appears to be important so the wearing of very tight underwear and trousers may be implicated in a low sperm count. Likewise radiation may damage the sperm-producing cells, the spermatocytes, and it is usual therefore for workers in atmospheres where there may be radiation (e.g. radiographers and radiologists in hospital radio-diagnostic departments) to wear protective lead aprons.

It is interesting to know that men with sedentary occupations – truck drivers, taxi drivers, office workers – tend to have lower average sperm counts than those employed in less sedentary jobs.

There is a condition known as *retrograde ejaculation* where the sperm pass back into the bladder at the time of ejaculation rather than down the urethra. The cause may be certain drugs such as tranquillisers or anti-hypertension therapy. The diagnosis is made by finding no sperm in the ejaculate but sperm in the urine instead. Where it seems to be a result of medication, changing the drug or reducing its dosage may improve the situation.

Otherwise sperm may have to be collected from the urine and used in artificial insemination (see Chapter 6, pp. 63–5).

Sexual problems such as *failure of erection* or *failure to maintain an erection* may be the basis of the male side of the problem of infertility. It is often assumed that these problems are either organic (as a result of neurological conditions such as multiple sclerosis, for example) or psychological. They often have a mixed cause and the association of erectile failure (or impotence as it is usually referred to) with drugs, the abuse of alcohol, other medical conditions such as diabetes as well as personal and marital problems must be remembered when investigations begin.

These then constitute the main background causes for male infertility and we shall see later how investigations are arranged, based on these background causes and how each cause is tackled and with what treatment.

## The female factor

Now let us look at where things can go wrong in the female partner. And in the same way, if we bear the facts of her anatomy and physiology (the way structures function) in mind we can map out where problems may arise.

### ABNORMAL ANATOMY

In order to achieve a pregnancy these structures are necessary – and they must function normally – ovaries, tubes, uterus, vagina.

*Absence or maldevelopment of organs*

Although not a common cause of infertility, nevertheless abnormalities of the development of the essential female organs may be found.

*Absence of a vagina* may be partial or complete but this will usually have been detected much earlier in a woman's life.

There are various rare conditions based on either chromosome or hormone abnormalities where abnormalities of sexual organ development occur. These, it must be emphasised, are rare and will usually be identified at a much earlier stage than we are discussing. For instance, in 'gonadal dysgenesis' (Turner's syndrome), there is loss of one X chromosome from the nucleus (so the individual is described as XO). The ovaries fail to develop beyond a 'streak' and at puberty there is failure of secondary sexual characteristics to develop. In an interesting variant of this (but again very rare) the chromosome complement may be XX/XO or XY/XO. In the former there may be few apparent stigmata but the ovaries will fail prematurely in the twenties or thirties leading to infertility of an irreversible kind. In the latter, one gonad is a testis and one a 'streak' only. As a result there is often insufficient of the hormone testosterone to counteract the natural female development.

The testis in such an individual has to be removed because of a high risk of becoming malignant. In any case the individual will have usually been brought up as a female and some masculinisation will occur at puberty from the male gonad so that to remove it becomes necessary for this reason. There will be no vagina (or just a pouch) and no uterus. With plastic surgery a new vagina can be fashioned and with female hormone therapy secondary female sexual characteristics (e.g. the breasts) are helped to develop. So, such an individual looks like, and can live like, a normal female but in the absence of a uterus can never conceive.

Rare hormone-based abnormalities are occasionally seen.

In '*congenital adrenal hyperplasia*' for instance there is an excess amount of the precursors of testosterone from the adrenal so that the female infant is exposed to excess of testosterone and is masculinised. The situation may be detected at birth but if not the baby will be brought up as a male (there is a big clitoris and fused labia mimicking a scrotum) and the true state of affairs not recognised until puberty.

There are several other developmental abnormalities which are variants of the above but they will not be discussed further in view of their rarity and the very small part they therefore play in our study of the background causes of failure to conceive.

Other maldevelopments of the genital tract which may be associated with infertility are (see Fig. 5/3, p. 56):

(a) *A vaginal septum*: Here a membrane of skin stretches across or up and down the vagina. The problem here is usually with achieving penetration at intercourse. Excision of the membrane is a comparatively simple surgical procedure. A transverse membrane at the level of the hymen is sometimes found in teenagers who present usually with failure to menstruate at an older age than expected. Because this is a complete membrane it blocks the outflow of menstrual blood and a state of *cryptomenorrhoea* (hidden menstruation) exists with the menstrual blood 'piling up' behind the membrane. Simple excision of the membrane drains the old blood and allows normal menstruation to take place. Although commoner than the other conditions discussed this tends to present in other ways than by failure to conceive.

(b) A variety of *developmental errors of the uterus* can occur because it develops from two halves which fuse together with the fusion junction breaking down to produce a single cavity. Rarely a cause of infertility in fact, these errors of development are more likely to be associated with recurring abortion or other problems such as premature labour and an abnormal lie of the baby in late pregnancy.

FUNCTIONAL DEFECTS

Here we come to the much commoner and more important aspects of failure to conceive in the female. From our basic knowledge we are going to have to consider the following.

Ovarian factors
Tubal factors
Uterine factors
Cervical factors
and, as always,
Miscellaneous factors

It must be also remembered that more than one cause may exist in the same individual.

*The ovarian factor*

Quite simply if the ovary does not function regularly – or at all – to produce eggs there will obviously be resultant infertility. We have seen how the stimulus to ovulation occurs so that we can understand the various situations which produce failure of the production of eggs.

1. *Premature ovarian failure*: Here the ovaries have simply stopped functioning at an earlier age than normally expected. This will be accompanied by failure to menstruate and is fortunately rare as it is irreversible.

*Secondary ovarian failure* may be the result of radiotherapy (*x*-ray therapy usually used for a malignancy) or surgery on the ovaries. In this latter case both ovaries may have been removed or such large areas excised that inadequate function remains in the portions left behind. These situations are fortunately also very rare.

2. *Hypothalamic-pituitary failure*: More commonly the ovary is capable of function and menstruation may be taking place but there is insufficient stimulus from the follicle stimulating

hormone (FSH) and luteinising hormone (LH) produced by the pituitary under the influence of the hypothalamus. These, as we have seen, are the hormones required for the maturation and development of an egg containing follicle in the ovary and its subsequent rupture and shedding of an egg.

Problems arising in the hypothalamus may be the result of anxiety and stress and are often associated with failure to menstruate also. Pituitary problems as such are tumour (called adenoma) which may be detected on special *x*-rays or are assumed (microadenoma) and are usually accompanied by a rise in the hormone prolactin and again frequently associated with amenorrhoea.

Problems in other glands of the body may affect the hypothalamic-pituitary system and either just occasional ovulation takes place or there is total shut-down – *anovulation*.

Malfunction of the adrenal or thyroid glands and the condition of diabetes are examples of other gland dysfunction influencing ovulation.

Another relatively recently recognised situation is called the '*inadequate luteal phase*' or '*luteal phase defect*'. Here ovulation occurs but maturation of the follicle and its conversion into a functioning corpus luteum is defective. True luteal phase deficiency is rare but a short luteal phase is not uncommon and may be associated with either infertility or very early miscarriages. A high prolactin level may be present in some.

### *Tubal factors*

Bearing in mind the structure and function of the Fallopian tubes we can readily understand that for the successful pick-up and transfer of the ovum, its subsequent fertilisation and continued transfer down the tube to the uterine cavity we need an undamaged tube preferably with intact fimbriae, an open tube, a tube that can move freely (mobile) and an intact lining membrane especially with undamaged specialised cells and their hair-like processes which waft the egg on its way.

The tube's entry into the uterus should also not be blocked.
What can go wrong?

1. *Infection* can distort the tube, pin it down to surrounding structures, damage its fimbriae, block its canal and destroy the specialised lining cells and their hair-like processes. Such infection is, unfortunately, not infrequently seen nowadays. Bacterial infection associated with abortion, the use of the coil or from surrounding structures such as appendicitis may result in damaged tubes. Gonococcal infection may be the cause and there are several other implicated organisms.

2. *Surgery* on the tubes may have been carried out in an attempt to open them up. Unfortunately although the tube may now be opened it has almost certainly lost its motility and its specialised lining cells will have been damaged. Obviously the operation of sterilisation either by excising a loop of tube or clipping it with a special device will occlude the tube. Surgery to reverse this operation tends to fail simply as a result of the scarring that the procedure itself then causes.

3. Other conditions may secondarily involve the tubes either by blocking them or causing adhesions which interfere with their function. Such a condition is *endometriosis* and as it is not infrequently associated with infertility and as a result a cause of great concern to the sufferer it is worth diverting our discussion for a moment to learn what exactly this condition is.

*Endometriosis*: The lining of the cavity of the uterus is called the endometrium and its specialised cells are the endometrial cells. For reasons that are unknown these endometrial cells are, in some women, found in other areas of the body. Chiefly they are sited in the pelvic cavity – on the floor of the pelvis, behind the uterus, on the ovaries, on the surface of the bladder in front of the uterus. More distant sites are in the bowel, the appendix, the umbilicus, the vagina and the scars of wounds on the abdomen especially where the surgery has been on the uterus, entering its cavity.

The appearance of these areas of endometriosis varies greatly from tiny black shiny spots (called, picturesquely, 'pheasants' eyes') to areas of puckering and scarring with adhesion of one organ to another (e.g. the ovary and tube stuck to the back of the uterus). In endometriosis of the ovary, cysts may develop reaching quite large sizes and filled with typical black tarry material which is old inspissated blood.

The symptoms produced by endometriosis can be understood when it is realised that these endometrial cells will respond to hormone changes as the endometrium itself does. They swell up and as menstruation occurs they 'crumble' too producing menstrual-like material around them. This is very irritating and dysmenorrhoea will result.

Not only that but the areas themselves will remain painful so that pain at times other than the periods is a feature and especially pain on pressure – e.g. dyspareunia – may be a major problem.

So far as the tubes are concerned endometriosis within the structure of the tube itself is rare but adhesions as a result of surrounding endometriosis may involve the tubes, preventing their normal functioning. It is also interesting to know that even without direct involvement of the tubes patients with scattered areas of endometriosis are not infrequently infertile. It is as if their reproductive apparatus has 'gone wrong' in some way ending up with both infertility *and* endometriosis: not a very scientific concept. Incidentally the condition is most common in women over 30 who have not had children.

Treatment of endometriosis may be surgical or medical. *Surgical* treatment in its most radical form would be removal of the uterus and the tubes and ovaries. This would only be used in older women with extensive endometriosis. Less radical surgery may be employed such as removal of endometriotic cysts and excision or diathermisation (burning, using electrocautery) of patches of endometriosis.

*Medical treatment* may be used as an adjunct to surgery or, once the diagnosis has been made and particularly with younger women and limited disease, as the treatment of choice. The contraceptive pill is of some value in treatment or the hormone progesterone alone may be more efficient. A more modern drug called danazol (Danol) is now the specific treatment. It is taken by mouth usually twice a day for a varying period of time, usually six to nine months. The periods are often suppressed during this time and the areas of endometriosis seem to 'melt' away. Its mode of action need not concern us here but in a general sense Danol is an 'antihormone'. If a pregnancy can be achieved after treatment (or before, of course) this is the treatment *par excellence* for endometriosis. Unfortunately it may recur after pregnancy.

Endometriosis is a curious condition affecting younger age groups but, as we have seen, with early diagnosis and adequate treatment it need not be a bar to conceiving.

*Uterine factors*

It is important to say that even the most misshapen uterus may carry a pregnancy successfully. However, early miscarriage may result from abnormalities of the shape of the cavity of the uterus such as are caused by fibroids which are benign tumours of the muscle of the uterus and which may protrude into the cavity grossly distorting it. In the absence of any other cause for infertility and where there are many fibroids present, surgery to remove these tumours and attempt to recreate a more normal uterus may be advisable.

Disease of the lining of the cavity, the endometrium, may prevent conception. Tuberculosis is such a condition but is rarely found in the West in the present day.

There is a rare condition called Asherman's syndrome where the cavity of the uterus is obliterated by the front and back walls being stuck together. This can follow curettage of the uterine cavity, perhaps followed by infection, but is an extremely uncommon situation.

It is true to say that uterine factors in infertility are not common in comparison with the other factors. Incidentally retroversion of the uterus (tilted backwards instead of the more usual forwards) is *not* a cause of failure to conceive.

*Cervical factors*

The neck of the womb, however, as distinct from the body and cavity of the womb, may play quite an important part in infertility.

In order for sperm to enter the uterus and get to the tubes to meet and fertilise the ovum they have first of all to penetrate the mucus – the sticky watery material – which plugs the cervix. Favourable mucus is thin and clear and capable of being drawn out into long threads (this is called 'spinnbarkeit') and the mucus is made favourable by the high oestrogen levels present just before ovulation. At other times in the cycle the mucus is thick and cloudy and tends to inhibit the movement of sperm.

In some women there is too little cervical mucus and naturally if they are not ovulating then it is too thick and sticky. Even if ovulation is taking place it is possible for the mucus to remain 'hostile' to sperm. This can be a result of infection or the presence of antibodies in the mucus. Antibodies are a feature of the body's normal defence mechanism to foreign cells – disease, infection, and so on. But the presence of antisperm antibodies can be a problem where a couple are attempting to conceive. This aspect of infertility will be discussed further later in the book.

*Miscellaneous factors*

Apart from these major causes of infertility which we have

outlined there are several 'lesser' contributory factors. When a couple are being investigated these factors must be remembered and are often simply checked by taking a careful detailed history and by a preliminary examination.

For instance if the woman has an infection of the vagina this may contribute to her failure to conceive and must be cleared up.

Then again problems of intercourse itself may become apparent. For instance, impotence in the man or failure to penetrate the vagina because of *vaginismus* in the woman. Vaginismus is an undue tightening and 'spasm' of the muscles of the vagina and may be due to fear or distaste of intercourse or to local conditions such as scarring or infection producing pain. It is quite possible for a pregnancy to result from sperm deposited on the vulva only but this is rare and penetration of the vagina with deposition of the sperm in the upper vagina is really a prerequisite for pregnancy. Just occasionally a couple may be ignorant of their anatomy and intercourse may indeed be taking place only between the labia or through the rectum. Education and sometimes sex therapy will be necessary to rectify this sort of situation.

The timing of intercourse is important in order to achieve a pregnancy. We have seen how in a 28-day cycle ovulation tends to occur about day 14. If intercourse never occurs around this time then the chances of achieving success are slender.

A surprising number of couples feel that when they have decided to start a family it will happen with no delay at all – and this sometimes when intercourse is not occurring very often or even when the husband is away for long stretches of time – for example in the Navy. Explanation and encouragement may be all that is required here.

This then has been a review of what can go wrong with the anatomy and physiology of both the male and the female partner to result in infertility. We can now move on logically to consider the investigations which will be initiated for the infertile couple based on these problems.

# 4

# Investigations for the Man

The following two chapters are to be concerned with the tests that are carried out to try and establish the reason – or reasons – for a couple's failing to conceive. The first chapter considers the male partner, the second the female. But right away let us realise that this is the wrong approach. It is convenient and logical to separate the male and female when writing about the problem of infertility but it must be stressed at the outset that the problem is a mutual one and that both partners should be interviewed together and examinations and investigations initiated at the same time.

The first step in investigation is to take a history from the couple. It has been suggested that this should be done separately so that facts can be corroborated and details revealed which may be confidential. This may be true but it is on the whole much more acceptable to a couple that they should share in the initial interview at least. Opportunity will arise later for the couple to be seen individually and if there are 'secrets' they can be revealed then.

What are the facts in a couple's history that are important? Here, in list form, are the main facts that will be queried and verified by the investigating doctor.

- The ages and occupations of the couple
- Any previous marriages?
- How long have they been married?
- How long was contraception used and what was the method?
- Have either had previous children or, in the case of a

woman, ever had a previous pregnancy of any duration?

- Has either had any previous illness or operation? In the case of the woman acute appendicitis, for example, is important since the near-by pelvic organs may have been secondarily involved in the infection. Any pelvic surgery is important. In the man's case mumps with its complication of orchitis is obviously important – or any other type of genital infection
- The family medical history on both sides
- Is intercourse painless; how often does it occur; do they know anything about the fertile period of the month?
- Is menstruation regular; is it painful or painless?

**Examination**

The next step in the investigation of an infertile couple is the general examination.

Such a couple will almost always first go to their own family doctor to seek help and advice and in that case general and local examination of both man and woman will be done. The gynaecologist, to whom the couple will ultimately be sent for specialised investigations, will normally confine his/her examination to the woman. Fundamentally the man's capacity for fertility rests on his sperm count and if this proves to be abnormal then the gynaecologist will refer him to the urologist – a specialist in genito-urinary medicine – and a more detailed examination of the man will be carried out.

However, to return to the initial examination, which should preferably be by the family doctor.

For both man and woman a general examination will first be carried out – general appearance, weight, colour, heart, lungs, blood pressure, and so on. Then the reproductive system will be looked at. In the case of the man, the penis, the testes, the epididymes, the prostate – these will all be examined for abnormalities.

Then in the woman's case the vulva, the vagina (is penetration taking place? is she displaying vaginismus even at examination?), the uterus (its size, regularity of outline, mobility) the tubes and ovaries (enlargement, fixity, undue tenderness) will all be carefully palpated and assessed.

These then are the preliminary general assessments of the infertile couple. Now we come to the more specialised detailed investigations. First, the male partner:

## ASSESSMENT OF MALE FERTILITY

### *Semen analysis*

The findings of a normal analysis have already been given (p. 28) but, to repeat, it is not just the numbers of sperm present that we are interested in it is also their movement, their shape and their appearance.

If an abnormal result is obtained then a second specimen will be looked at, as we have mentioned, before any conclusions are drawn.

Another aspect of the semen specimen which is looked at is the total volume, which is normally 1–4ml. Of course the amount may be reduced simply because of the difficulty a man may find in producing the specimen and this must be taken into account. Again the liquefaction and viscosity are of some importance. When ejaculated, semen is liquid but coagulates almost immediately. Within 10 to 20 minutes it has liquefied again but remains viscous. If the semen does not liquefy sperm are not able to achieve normal motility and equally if there is excessive viscosity the sperm become clumped together and cannot become motile.

If the male partner is unable to produce a specimen of semen then a post-coital test will be done. This test, however, is complementary to the semen analysis and will be part of the examination in any case. It will be described under the female investigations.

*Hormone investigations*

If an abnormality is found in the sperm count then, as we have seen, a full examination will be carried out usually by a urologist. Blood may be taken to check the relevant hormone levels especially testosterone and FSH. A high level of the latter hormone from the pituitary points to testicular damage. In the presence of azoospermia (no sperm in the semen sample) a normal level would indicate obstruction to the passage of sperm.

Low values of FSH, LH and testosterone may indicate a problem in the pituitary gland itself.

The hormone prolactin may be measured. A high level, indicating a prolactin secreting tumour of the pituitary or disorder of the hypothalamus, may result in oligospermia (reduced sperm numbers).

*Chromosome studies*

These will be carried out if there are other stigmata of abnormal or immature development. We have already seen how a chromosome abnormality, such as Klinefelter's syndrome, will be associated with azoospermia and testicular failure.

*Biopsy of the testes*

Under certain circumstances this may be recommended but with increasing knowledge of the correlation of hormone levels to the various causes of male infertility this procedure is not so often carried out nowadays.

*Biochemistry of the semen*

Measurement of substances such as acid phosphatase, fructose and carnitine – and their presence or absence in the semen – may give a further clue as to the source of the problem of oligo- or azoospermia.

*Immunological tests*

The understanding of the immunology of infertility is a developing aspect of the problem. One very new and exciting area is discussed in the section on recurrent abortion (see p. 79).

Antibodies to sperm can be demonstrated in the blood of either the woman or the man himself. Auto-antibodies may be present also in seminal plasma. Unfortunately, as yet, treatment is unsatisfactory.

Where antibodies are demonstrated in the mucus of the cervix, shown by immobilisation of the partner's sperm, this can sometimes be helped by the partner using a sheath for a time to prevent contact. By-passing the cervical mucus

**Table 4/1** Male infertility: causes and investigations

| *Causes* | *Investigations* |
|---|---|
| Control of testicular function | Hormone measurements |
| Abnormalities of the testes | History, e.g. chronic illness<br>Examination<br>Chromosome studies<br>Biopsy |
| Obstruction to ducts | History: trauma<br>surgery<br>infection<br>Examination |
| Infection | Semen analysis/culture<br>Examination, e.g. prostate |
| Coital difficulties, e.g. impotence | History<br>Examination |
| Psychological problems | History |
| Immunological problems | Antibody measurements in semen or blood |

through artificial insemination is another way round this problem.

A great deal remains to be elucidated on the subject of immunology in relation to both male and female infertility.

In spite of the availability of these investigations we are sometimes left with male 'idiopathic' infertility, that is where there is oligo- or azoospermia with no detectable cause for it.

It may be helpful to summarise the basic causes of male infertility indicating the tests/investigations employed for each (Table 4/1). These are fundamentally based on the finding first of all of an abnormal semen sample. Another fundamental fact must be stressed at this point, however, and that is that a normal result does not necessarily mean that a man is fertile. As one authority has put it 'seminal analysis can seldom be relied upon to indicate definite infertility in the male and never to indicate definite fertility'. Other links in the chain of male fertility remain to be identified in the future.

# 5

# Investigations for the Woman

The fact that the infertile couple should be investigated in parallel cannot be repeated often enough. We have already discussed the history that should be obtained from them and the preliminary examination carried out on each. It goes without saying (in spite of the proviso in the last chapter) that if a normal semen sample is obtained then the investigations for the woman should be pursued. If, however, there is an abnormal sample then apart from simple 'non-invasive' investigations the women's testing will be deferred until the veracity of, or basis for, the abnormal semen sample is established.

We have already considered the steps in assessing male fertility. For the female we can follow the same logical approach remembering what we have learned about the anatomy and physiology of female fertility. As with any medical problem we start with the history and examination and the important points to be looked for in this respect in the female have already been considered

## Assessment of female fertility

Having obtained the history from the woman and completed a general and pelvic examination as previously outlined we now consider the special investigations which will be carried out. Basically we are going to check that the woman is ovulating (producing eggs), that the tubes are open and healthy so that a sperm can get to the egg and that, once fertilised, the egg can travel down to the uterus, that the uterus is capable of allowing implantation. We must also check that the sperm is able to gain access to the uterus and tube.

Table 5/1 gives a summary of the steps in investigation each of which we will then study in a little more detail.

**Table 5/1** Female infertility: a summary of investigations

History

General and local examination

Special investigations

| *Ovulation* | *Tubal patency* | *Uterine and cervical factors* |
|---|---|---|
| Basal temperature | Insufflation | D and C |
| Blood progesterone | *x*-ray hysterosalpingogram | Hysterogram |
| Endometrial biopsy | Laparoscopy | Cervical mucus |
| Ultrasound | | Post-coital test |
| | | Antibody testing |

OVULATION

Fundamental to achieving a pregnancy is the production of eggs. Regular menstruation generally implies regular ovulation – but not always, so it is mandatory in the apparently infertile woman to check whether ovulation is taking place. The simplest method is to get her to keep a temperature chart and this is demonstrated in Figure 5/1.

(a) Typically a woman's basal temperature (taken first thing in the morning before getting out of bed or taking any food or fluid) varies in the two phases of her monthly cycle as we can see from Figure 5/1. In the first half – or proliferative phase – it is low and on the day before ovulation a drop occurs then a

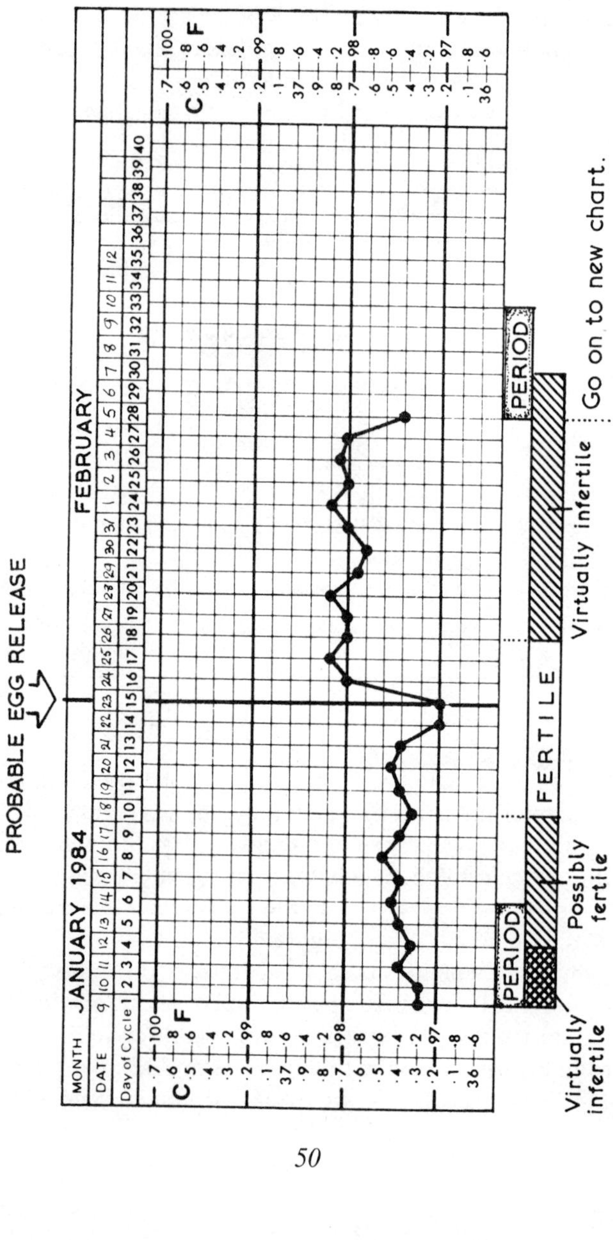


Fig. 5/1 A basal temperature chart showing ovulation

rise above the previous baseline on the day after. This rise continues for the next 2–4 days reaching a plateau and finally 1–3 days before menstruation there is a fall to levels seen in the proliferative phase.

This is a relatively simple method of monitoring cycles to see if they are ovulatory and together with the change in cervical mucus (see p. 39) can provide a 'do-it-yourself' method for the couple. Unfortunately it has several drawbacks. It is for instance unreliable, it is limited in the information it gives and, perhaps worst of all, it has the danger of making the couple neurotic and of destroying spontaneity in their married life.

So although it is a useful complement to other investigations, used for a few cycles only, we have to turn to more sophisticated methods for demonstrating ovulation.

(b) The level of the hormone progesterone in the middle of the luteal phase is probably the most reliable method of checking ovulation and a blood specimen taken between day 19–21 after the onset of menstruation will be arranged.

(c) The change which takes place in the lining of the cavity of the uterus (the endometrium) after ovulation has occurred is another means of identifying ovulation. We have already seen how the endometrium becomes much thicker, filled with glands, full of secretion and with a rich blood supply. This appearance only occurs if ovulation has taken place so that by taking a strip of endometrium in the second half of a cycle definite proof of ovulation can be obtained.

A curettage (scraping out the endometrium) can be performed therefore for checking ovulation but in fact nowadays, with most laboratories able to carry out progesterone level measurements, it is not so often used as a diagnostic procedure.

Obviously, if it is to be carried out, then some form of contraception (barrier is best, either the cap or the sheath) should be used since there is always the possibility (however remote) of conception occurring in that cycle.

(d) The use of ultrasound to monitor the development of a follicle is a technique which is proving to be increasingly popular and reliable.

Figure 5/2 shows the appearance of a follicle just prior to ovulation. At the time of writing, this technique is used particularly in monitoring cycles where for instance in vitro fertilisation is being used and it is essential to identify the exact time to 'harvest' the egg. Cycles in which drug stimulation of ovulation is being employed can also be monitored in this way.

Hopefully, with increasing expertise in ultrasonography and its interpretation the method will be used more and more to check ovulation

### TUBAL PATENCY

It goes without saying that to achieve conception not only must there be an egg available but one if not both of the Fallopian tubes should be open and have normal function. That function, you will remember, is motility of the muscular walls and intact lining cells and their cilia so that the sperm can reach the ovum and, once fertilised, the egg can be wafted down to the uterine cavity.

If ovulation is shown to be occurring satisfactorily, then tubal patency will be checked next (after the semen analysis, of course). If an individual's history suggests previous pelvic infection or there have been conditions such as an acute appendicitis which might have produced associated tubal infection then assessment of the tube will be arranged at an early stage.

What are the methods used to check the tubes?

(a) *Insufflation of the tubes*

This is an older method not frequently employed nowadays probably because it is regarded as unreliable although it does

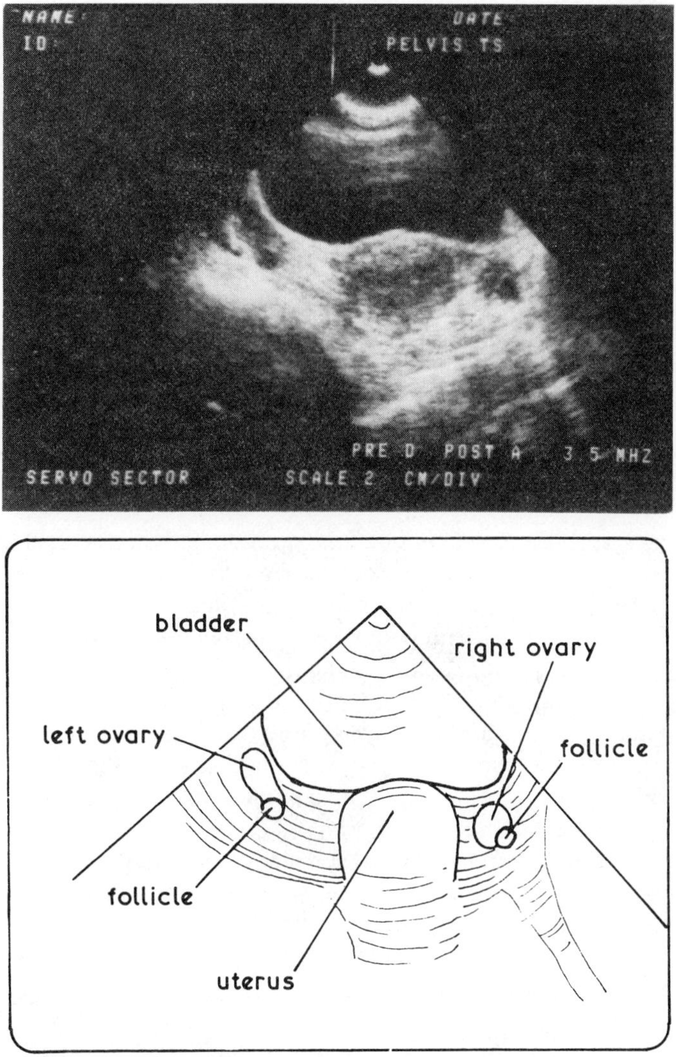


Fig. 5/2 *Above* Ultrasound scan showing follicles in ovaries
*Below* Line drawing to show relevant features

have the benefit of simplicity and relative non-invasiveness. Known as Rubin's test it consists of passing carbon dioxide gas through the cervix into the uterine cavity and, if they are patent, through the tubes. The pressure at which the gas passes can be recorded – it rises at first then drops as the gas escapes from the tubes. The gas can be heard escaping from the tubes through a stethoscope placed on each side of the lower abdomen.

The procedure may be done without an anaesthetic but in practice, particularly if the patient being investigated has never been pregnant before, a general anaesthetic will be required.

(b) *Hysterosalpingography*

In this test a radio-opaque material is passed through the cervix into the uterine cavity and so into the tubes. Because it is radio-opaque its progress can be followed on an *x*-ray viewing box. If the tubes (or one tube) are blocked then no spill of the injected substance will be seen from the ends of the tubes.

All sites of blockage can be detected whether at the end of the tube, just as it enters the uterus, or at a point in between, so the test is valuable in locating the problem area.

The other important aspect of the test – implied in the name *hystero*salpingography – is that the shape, size and outline of the uterine cavity can be studied as well as the tubes. This may be of some importance in the investigation of infertility as we shall see.

Like Rubin's test, hysterosalpingography may be carried out with, or without, general anaesthetic. Nowadays, although perhaps no longer the first choice of investigation, the procedure is still commonly employed often as a complement to laparoscopy.

(c) *Laparoscopy*

This method of investigation has revolutionised the investigation of the infertile patient. In it, a long narrow telescope is passed into the abdominal cavity through a tiny incision just under the navel. By distending the abdominal cavity with carbon dioxide gas first, a clear view of the uterus and tubes is obtained. A mixture of methylene blue dye and saline is injected through the cervix and can be watched through the laparoscope as it progresses along the tubes and spills out at the ends.

The value of this method of investigation lies in the fact that not only can the tubes' patency be checked but their overall appearance inspected and the presence of other conditions of the pelvis which may be relevant, spotted.

Most authorities would use 'laparoscopy and instillation of dye', as it is described, as the first line in investigation of tubal function

### UTERINE AND CERVICAL FACTORS

We have already mentioned the *x*-ray procedure of hysterosalpingography as playing a part in the investigation of infertility. Such abnormalities as deformity of the *uterine* cavity by fibroids, (for example) can be picked up. It is, however, doubtful that such problems are a cause of infertility; rather may they result in recurrent miscarriages. Nevertheless it is necessary to know that the uterine cavity is normal in shape and capable of 'holding' a fertilised egg.

Curettage has already been mentioned as playing a part in infertility investigations mainly by securing pieces of endometrium for laboratory examination. The instrument used, the curette, can demonstrate any irregularities of the cavity.

We have already mentioned the very rare condition called Asherman's syndrome where the front and back walls of the uterus become adherent to each other thereby obliterating the uterine cavity. This can result from over-vigorous curettage but is indeed rare and results not only in infertility but also in absence of menstruation. If suspected the problem can be diagnosed by a hysterogram or by the use of ultrasound.

Various malformations of the uterus may depress fertility although again they may be more associated with recurrent miscarriages. For interest, a few such malformations are shown in Figure 5/3. Again they are rare but will be demonstrated by the hysterogram or by ultrasound in some cases.

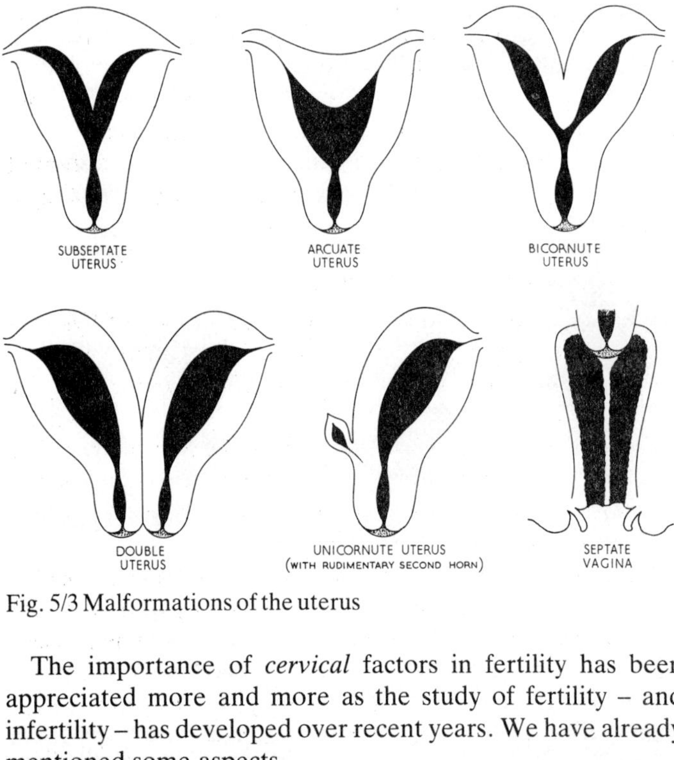


Fig. 5/3 Malformations of the uterus

The importance of *cervical* factors in fertility has been appreciated more and more as the study of fertility – and infertility – has developed over recent years. We have already mentioned some aspects.

So far as the structure of the cervix is concerned we ought to consider for a moment the problem of *cervical incompetence*. This will be discussed later in considering recurrent abortions but briefly it implies that the neck of the womb is slack, especially at the *internal os* – the opening into the womb itself – and is therefore incompetent to 'hold on to' a pregnancy. While it is possible that such a situation would mean that even the earliest fertilised egg would not be retained in the uterine cavity, in practice pregnancies can get started but will abort ultimately (usually after 14 weeks) when they begin to extrude through the incompetent cervix.

More important in our study of infertility are the functional aspects of the cervix. When the sperm enter the uterus the first barrier they meet is the cervical mucus, the sticky substance secreted by the glands of the cervix. To be favourable to receive the sperm the mucus has to be thin and clear and can be drawn out into long threads (a property known as spinnbarkeit). If spread out on a glass slide it shows the appearance of 'ferning'. All these appearances are associated with ovulation so that every preparation is being made to 'help' the sperm reach the egg produced at that time. At other times in the monthly cycle the mucus is thick and sticky and inhibits the passage of sperm (nature's somewhat inadequate attempt at 'natural' contraception). The changes in the mucus at the time of ovulation are due to a rise in the hormone oestrogen.

Now hostility of the sperm may arise as a result of infection or the presence of antibodies as we have already mentioned. To test the compatibility, or suitability, of the cervical mucus for the passage of sperm the *post-coital test* is carried out.

### *The post-coital test*

The test is carried out at mid-cycle within 12 hours of intercourse following 4 or 5 days of refraining from intercourse. A sample of mucus is aspirated from the cervical canal – quite simply done during a routine vaginal examination – and examined under the microscope. Its quantity, spinnbarkeit quality and stickiness are first assessed then it is spread out on a glass slide and examined. In a normal situation at least

5 motile sperm per high power field (hpf) should be seen. These show progressive motion and in an abnormal situation either no sperm will be seen or only one or two which are inactive.

More sophisticated tests can be carried out, for example the *sperm hostility test*. If, on a post-coital test as described above, a few sperm are seen which are immotile this test may be done. Essentially what happens is that a specimen of mid-cycle mucus is brought into contact with a specimen of sperm and the penetration of the sperm into the mucus examined under the microscope.

More elaboration of this simple test may be done where the semen is brought into contact with donor mucus or donor semen brought into contact with the cervical mucus being tested. In this way it is possible to test whether the problem rests with the mucus, sperm or indeed technique of coitus.

Needless to say infection of the cervix will be identified and appropriately treated during the course of investigations.

These then are the investigations for the female partner checking her ability to produce eggs, the patency and function of her tubes to transport them, the normality of the uterus to receive a fertilised egg and the healthiness and suitability of the cervical mucus to allow passage of the sperm to trigger off the whole mechanism of conception. Having looked at the investigations and identified where faults may arise we must now consider what can be done to rectify these faults.

# 6

# Treatment for the Man

We have already stressed the need to investigate both partners concurrently. If a fault is found in one then it should be corrected (if possible) before elaborate and possibly invasive investigations are carried out on the other partner. It has also been shown that the man's potential fertility will be demonstrated by a normal semen analysis – the simplest of tests to carry out. Note, however, that the phrase used was 'potential fertility' – just because a man has a normal semen analysis does not mean that he is definitely fertile although more often than not it does.

If, in the course of the investigation of a poor semen analysis a problem is found requiring either elaborate medical therapy or an attempt at intricate surgery, then before embarking on these the female partner should first of all be shown to be 'normal'.

In looking at the treatment available for male fertility or sub-fertility we can logically follow the problems outlined in Chapter 3 and see what can be done to rectify these problems.

## 1. Anatomical abnormalities

If the physical difficulty is *hypospadias* with the urethral opening on the under surface of the penis surgery may be possible. Even after corrective surgery, however, the deposition of sperm in the upper vagina may still not occur. In this case artificial insemination may be necessary. We shall examine the whole question of artificial insemination at the end of this chapter.

Simpler anatomical abnormalities may exist such as tight foreskin or phimosis and are more amenable to surgery.

*Cryptorchidism* where one or both testes are undescended into the scrotum, although rarely found in adult life, requires surgery. Normally such a situation is recognised in infancy and the operation to bring down the undescended testis, known as orchidopexy, is advisable by the fifth birthday. If this problem is found in an infertility clinic then the type of operation required depends on the size of the testis involved. If it is very small (and no spermatogenesis will be occurring in such an organ) then the best thing is to remove it altogether. Lying in the groin, such an undescended testis may give pain, is liable to injury and worse still seems to be prone to malignant change. So since it is of no value it is better removed. If, however, it is a good size (greater than 3cm in length or 10ml in volume) then it is worth bringing it down into the scrotum by the procedure of orchidopexy and just occasionally spermatogenesis will begin. Certainly such a testis will have an endocrine function and produce the male hormone.

Where *genetic abnormalities* are detected such as Klinefelter's syndrome with abnormal chromosomes nothing can be done and here the question of artificial insemination by a donor will have to be considered. This will be discussed later.

Adoption is another possibility that must always be held in reserve for such situations where absolute infertility is demonstrated. Unfortunately it is true to say that facilities for adoption are not as easy as they once were.

Another anatomical abnormality which we have mentioned is *absence of the vas deferens – absence of the epididymis* may also occur. Operations have been devised for the construction or implantation of an artificial reservoir from which spermatozoa may be collected and insemination carried out. But such procedures have not proved to be very successful in practice even though they may sound an attractive proposition in theory.

*Varicocele* is a much more common problem. Here the varicosities round the epididymis and vas deferens depress spermatogenesis possibly by creating an unsuitably high local temperature. The operation required is to ligate (tie off) the varicocele just as one ties off varicose veins in the legs. The operation to ligate the varicocele was at one time regarded as the most successful method of treatment for the infertile male and it was almost a relief to find a varicocele as it were, so that something active could be done.

Now it is realised that not all varicoceles need surgery and various tests such as special *x*-rays may be done first to assess the need for operation. If a very low sperm count is found – or azoospermia – and abnormalities of the internal spermatic vein demonstrated then surgery is worthwhile. In doubtful cases other causes of infertility must be looked for first.

## 2. Functional defects

We have seen how testicular function is controlled by the brain (its hypothalamus) through the pituitary gland. Disease or malfunction of these areas or associated endocrine glands will lead to depression or total inhibition of spermatogenesis.

Disease of the *thyroid* or *adrenal glands* may lead to low fertility and must be treated in their own right. Improvement in fertility may well result.

*High prolactin levels* may be detected and in men these cause malfunction of the gonads. Treatment with the drug bromocriptine which depresses the prolactin level will restore function.

There may be pituitary disease or rare conditions of the hypothalamus. As a result the production of gonadotrophins ceases, the testes get smaller, the production of FSH and LH fails. In these rare problems gonadotrophin therapy can be given and the sperm count will slowly improve.

Other gonadal stimulants are used but the results are often

disappointing. One such drug is clomiphene. Testosterone itself is given by some clinicians. During therapy spermatogenesis is actually depressed but there was thought to be a rebound effect when treatment was discontinued and the production of sperm greatly improved. This is no longer believed to be the case and the only reason nowadays for giving testosterone is where there is a problem of poor libido.

In the individual there may be primary testicular failure which is absolute. The diagnosis is made by the finding of small testes and a very elevated FSH level. No treatment is possible and only artificial insemination by a donor or adoption can be offered.

We have seen how the mumps virus and other infections such as gonorrhoea or non-specific bacterial infections can damage the testes and their function to a greater or lesser degree. The damage is irreversible in most instances.

Active infection of the genital tract may affect the viscosity and liquefaction of the semen and treatment with antibiotics may effect improvement. Prolonged therapy with antibiotics known to be secreted into the seminal fluid, such as erythromycin, tetracycline and cephalosporin, is employed and success claimed.

We have seen how drugs may affect testicular function and this will include excess alcohol and possibly nicotine abuse. The answer to these problems is obvious.

Anti-cancer chemotherapy suppresses sperm production and where such treatment is necessary banking of the sperm beforehand should be offered where conception is likely to be sought later.

A number of other miscellaneous factors were mentioned in considering abnormalities of function of the testes. For example the environmental temperature of the testes is important and men with low sperm counts should be advised to wear loose underwear and avoid tight jeans for instance. Testicular cooling may be helpful and spraying the testes with cold water morning and evening has been recommended. For men with sedentary jobs these points plus plenty of exercise when possible may improve a low sperm count.

Where *retrograde ejaculation* occurs – diagnosed by finding sperm in the urine rather than in the semen – then sperm may be obtained from the urine and used for artificial insemination. It may be necessary to re-suspend the sperm in a medium more suitable than urine.

Retrograde ejaculation must be investigated and a cause found if possible. It may, for instance, be due to incompetence of the neck of the bladder and therefore surgical correction of this may be possible. Certain drugs may produce the problem and should be discontinued or alternatives found.

Correction of retrograde to 'antegrade' ejaculation may be achieved by teaching the man to contract his pelvic floor muscles at the time of orgasm. Another (uncomfortable) trick is to ejaculate with the bladder full. Some drugs, e.g. desipramine, are sometimes successful.

Sexual problems such as failure of erection or failure to maintain an erection may be psychologically based but disease must be excluded first, especially neurological disorders. The psychosomatic/psychosexual factors in infertility will be considered at the end of the next chapter.

## Artificial insemination

It seems appropriate to consider this at the conclusion of the section on treatment for male infertility.

The reasons for resorting to this method are, broadly, failure to achieve adequate coitus (impotence, retrograde or premature ejaculation), infertility in the male or familial disease on the husband's side.

There are two types of insemination, one where the husband's semen is used and the other where donor semen is used. The first method will be employed where there are coital difficulties but a fertile male, the second where there is azoospermia or virtually so.

Some clinicians adopt wider criteria for the use of artificial insemination believing that by taking sperm and placing it directly on to the cervix or even into the uterus there is a greater chance of success. On the whole, however, this is probably not so.

### TECHNIQUE

The semen is collected in a special container by masturbation and is transferred into the upper vagina or cervical canal as soon as possible (within 2 hours). This procedure must be done at the time of ovulation and this is monitored by checking the cervical mucus, measuring LH levels and in some centres watching the growth of the dominant follicle in the ovary by ultrasound scanning. Timing may be made more exact by the use of a simple fertility drug such as clomiphene. The procedure of insemination should be carried out for two or three days consecutively during the fertile period. This is one of the reasons why sperm 'banks' may be used with a collection of the husband's semen kept frozen at about −190°C in liquid nitrogen. On thawing, the sperm are active and capable of fertilisation even after long periods of storage.

The semen specimen is either injected on to the cervical external os using a fine glass pipette or syringe, or the specimen can be put into a cervical cap and placed over the cervix.

The simplest method is to put the semen into the upper vagina and this method can easily be used by the woman herself although she can also be taught to use the cervical cap.

Several sessions of insemination over several cycles are usually required before success is achieved.

### INSEMINATION BY A DONOR (AID)

Where there are the coital difficulties described there is usually no difficulty in a couple's accepting the idea of artificial insemination using the husband's semen. When it comes to the idea of using donor semen it is a different matter altogether and one which many couples find totally unacceptable.

The technique is used where the woman is fertile but the male is not. Choice of donors must be a careful one – no personal history of disease or inherited familial disorders, the semen free of infection, the anonymity of the donor must be maintained and so on.

Often 'banks' of frozen donor sperm are kept in clinics where a lot of this work is done. The ethical and legal aspects of such techniques are complicated. While ethically acceptable in this country nevertheless some clinicians will not agree to carry out AID.

The legal situation is confused in that strictly speaking the child of AID is illegitimate. In the event there is no obligatory notification of AID and such a child is registered in the normal way.

Adoption is frequently chosen as an acceptable alternative to AID. Because the demand for babies greatly exceeds their availability this process in itself has become difficult, prolonged and not infrequently ends in disappointment.

It is said that where the woman of a couple is fertile, the difficulties of adoption are such that more couples are turning to the idea of AID.

In this chapter we have seen how each recognisable cause of infertility in the male can be tackled and treated often with great success. Many authorities are less than optimistic about the successful management of the infertile male but this may not be entirely justified. Surgery plays a small part, drugs may become of increasing importance. Unfortunately nothing as yet can be done to help the male in whom the basic production of sperm is absent. But it must be emphasised that this is a comparatively rare situation.

# 7

# Treatment for the Woman

Now we come to consider the treatment that is at present available for treating the infertile woman. Like the previous chapter we shall follow the headings outlined in Chapter 3 when we looked at the causes of female infertility. Basically that means that we shall examine how we can rectify faults in the ovary and ovulation, faults in the tubes, faults in implantation in the uterus and faults in the cervix and its environment.

### 1. Faults in the ovary – anovulation

Obviously if no eggs are being produced then there is no possibility of a pregnancy. Usually anovulation is associated with scanty infrequent periods or no periods at all – amenorrhoea – but not always. We have seen that it is important to check all infertile women, even although menstruation may be taking place quite regularly, for evidence of ovulation.

If it is clearly demonstrated that ovulation is not taking place but follicles are available which are capable of being fertilised (assessed by ultrasound and/or measuring hormone levels) then medical induction of ovulation can be attempted. In some cases the problem lies not so much in the ovulation but more in the immediately following phase, the luteal phase. Maintenance of an adequately functioning corpus luteum is necessary for conception and it is now recognised that a 'luteal deficiency' is a cause of infertility (in about 20 per cent of cases). Measurement of the progesterone level on or about day 19–21 is important in both anovulation and luteal deficiency.

The drugs used in inducing ovulation are now discussed.

(a) CLOMIPHENE CITRATE (CLOMID)

This drug is commonly used to produce ovulation. Its action is complex but basically it acts on the hypothalamic-pituitary system resulting in the production of increased amounts of FSH and LH which, as we have seen, stimulate the development of follicles. The tablets are taken (usually just one 50mg tablet to begin with) daily for 5 days starting either on the first day of menstruation or the third or sometimes the fifth day, depending on the specialist concerned. Whether ovulation occurs or not will be monitored by the patient's temperature chart or by arranging a day-19 blood progesterone level. The dose is increased if necessary. Ovulation occurs 8–10 days after the end of the course.

The drug is singularly free of side-effects although occasionally hot flushes, palpitations, visual blurring and abdominal discomfort can occur. An alternative drug with similar action is tamoxifen.

Ovulation is achieved in, it is said, 90 per cent of cases but with only a 40 per cent pregnancy rate.

Sometimes it may be decided to use other agents along with Clomid. Such a drug is HCG (human chorionic gonadotrophin) which if given about 7 days *after* the course of clomiphene may help to trigger off ovulation.

(b) GONADOTROPHINS

This is a more sophisticated and complex method of stimulating ovulation and must only be used where strict laboratory control is available.

Human menopausal gonadotrophin (HMG) contains FSH and LH and develops the follicle. HCG given afterwards provides the surge of LH required to produce ovulation. The woman receiving such treatment has to have frequent checks of oestrogen levels (in blood and urine) to see if the HMG has produced a satisfactory (but not excessive) response. The ovulation rate of this regime is 80 per cent – again a smaller rate for pregnancy of 50–55 per cent.

With the use of Clomid, multiple pregnancy, especially twins, is a possibility (15–25 per cent); with gonadotrophin therapy it is a real risk (over 50 per cent if monitoring is not very carefully carried out). Another risk of gonadotrophin therapy is excessive stimulation of the ovaries with cyst formation and in the worst cases 'blowing up' of the ovaries producing acute abdominal pain. It is because of this that it is felt that such therapy is probably best carried out at specialised centres. Monitoring is carried out by blood or urine testing of oestrogen samples and also now by the use of ultrasound scanning which can detect developing follicles.

(c) GONADOTROPHIN RELEASING HORMONE (GnRH)

The end result of this therapy is to encourage the production of FSH and LH. It is a newer type of therapy and those suitable for it must be chosen carefully and monitored by a specialist centre. Pulsed doses are given at 90-minute intervals and the equipment for injecting subcutaneously can be worn by the patient in the form of a small box not much bigger than a cigarette packet.

(d) BROMOCRIPTINE

If failure to ovulate has been shown to be due to a high level of the hormone prolactin then the drug which will reduce the level is bromocriptine. There are some side-effects of this drug to begin with – dizziness, nausea sometimes – so it is given in small doses at first increasing gradually to an effective dose. The effectiveness of the drug can be monitored by measuring prolactin levels in the blood but as menstruation has usually ceased with high levels of prolactin it will be restored as the prolactin level falls. Care must be taken to stop the drug as soon as a pregnancy has been achieved.

(e) PROGESTERONE

Another problem which may be detected in the endocrine investigation of the infertile woman is, as we have seen, an 'inadequate luteal phase'. This means that the second half of the cycle is either of too short a length or the progesterone produced is in too small a quantity. Oestrogen and progesterone measurements during the cycle will pinpoint this defect and either Clomid is given (if oestrogen level on or about day 12 is low) or progesterone during the luteal phase (if oestrogen level is good and follicle development adequate).

All these hormone considerations are complex and often confusing to the patient concerned. Measurement of hormone levels and often scanning of the ovaries using ultrasound may have to be done at frequent intervals throughout a cycle so as to get a clear picture of what is going on (or not, as the case may be). Only then can rational treatment be planned and, when it is given, equally intensive monitoring may be required to assess the efficacy of the treatment. Needless to say it seems a long drawn-out process (to the patient) and much patience is required. To understand at least to some extent what is happening helps.

## 2. Treatment of problems of tubal patency

First it should be emphasised that if one tube is shown to be open and apparently 'free' and therefore capable of normal function surgery should not be attempted on the other blocked tube. Surgery always has the possibility of adhesions (where one structure sticks to another, either because of some inflammation after surgery, or as a result of oozing of blood at the time of surgery) and the healthy tube may become 'damaged' as a result.

SURGICAL TECHNIQUES

Surgery on blocked tubes is of varying degrees depending on

the problem. If, for example, the tubes are simply 'fixed' and stuck down by adhesions all that may be required is to divide the adhesions, and free the tubes – the operation of *salpingolysis*. Opening up the tubes that are blocked may be necessary – a comparatively simple procedure if the blockage is at the distal end of the tube, the operation of *salpingostomy*. Or a wedge of blocked tube can be cut out and the two open ends of tube re-united – the operation of *neosalpingostomy* (not so easy to do and not so effective).

If the blockage is at the insertion of the tube into the uterus then the outer patent part of the tube can be cut away and reimplanted into the uterus – *tubal reimplantation*.

Traditionally these operations are done in a standard way, the gynaecologist working by naked eye. In recent years the technique of *microsurgery* has been introduced. This means that the gynaecologist is working with the help of a microscope to visualise details of the tubes and their blood vessels. This has made the surgery overall more successful but on the whole results are still disappointing. Success rates vary with the procedure required and are obviously reduced the more elaborate the surgery necessary. Results varying from 1 to 70 per cent are reported. The success of a particular procedure is not only influenced by which procedure has to be used but by the state of the tubes before surgery. For example, a tube that has been the site of previous infection is likely to have a damaged lining mucous membrane (which cannot be restored) and so although it may be opened up by surgery its function is not normal.

Better claims for success are made for the operation to restore tubal patency after the operation of sterilisation. This can really only be attempted if clips have been put on the tubes and that a relatively small area of clipped tube can then be excised and the ends re-anastomosed. Claims of 70 to 90 per cent are made but this is by no means the rule and it is still better to regard the operation of sterilisation as irreversible.

IN VITRO FERTILISATION (IVF)

In vitro fertilisation – or the 'test-tube' baby – is, in many ways, replacing surgery with its doubtful outcome for blocked tubes. Because of wide media publicity the basic principle of such a procedure is well known. The fundamental steps are:

(a) To stimulate the ovary with Clomid and monitor follicle development by ultrasound;
(b) To 'harvest', i.e. aspirate, one or more mature ova using laparoscopy or by a technique whereby the instruments are guided by ultrasonic control;
(c) To fertilise these ova in the laboratory using the husband's (or, if necessary, donor's) sperm and to culture the fertilised ovum;
(d) To transfer the now growing egg and implant it into the uterus previously primed with hormones so that its lining endometrium is in a receptive state.

Several attempts at monthly intervals may be required. It is obvious that such a technique needs very specialised equipment, laboratory facilities and skilled personnel and is therefore expensive. At the time of writing most of these centres are in the private hospital sector but a few National Health hospitals are beginning to run 'IVF programmes'.

GAMETE INTRA-FALLOPIAN TRANSFER

A recent variation is what is called GIFT – gamete intra-Fallopian transfer. This means taking active normal sperm and placing them directly in the Fallopian tube to meet the ovum. In other words fertilisation takes place 'in vivo' instead of 'in vitro'.

**3. Uterine factors**

Problems within the uterus itself have already been

described. Fibroids if they are thought to be significant in a problem of infertility may be removed by the operation of *myomectomy* which means 'shelling out' the fibroids and then reconstituting the uterus.

The rare condition of Asherman's syndrome has been described where the walls of the uterus become adherent thereby obliterating the cavity. This problem can be dealt with by insertion of a coil for some time.

Other abnormalities of uterine development and shape if they are considered to contribute to infertility can be dealt with by suitable corrective surgery.

## 4. Cervical factors

We have seen that mucus favourable to the passage of sperm is thin, clear and shows the quality of spinnbarkeit (drawing out into long threads). If smeared on a glass slide it appears as a fern pattern. These changes are all due to high oestrogen levels and in fact the mucus is at its most favourable 12–36 hours before ovulation when the level of oestrogen is high. This happens so that the sperm can gain access to the uterus and through to the tube ready to receive the ovum when it is shed from the ovary.

Infection may be a cause of altering the favourableness of the mucus and when detected should be treated – antibiotics for active infection (or other drugs depending on the organisms found) and cauterisation for the 'unhealthy' inflamed cervix.

Apparent hostility of cervical mucus to sperm can be dealt with in several ways. For example, oestrogen tablets may be given for a few days prior to expected ovulation. In some instances where sperm antibodies are suspected it may be appropriate for the male to use a sheath for a few months after which time sperm penetration may be found to have improved.

As we have already seen it is in these cases that artificial insemination may be advisable.

### 5. Miscellaneous factors

During the course of investigation other factors may be found which may contribute to the problem of delayed fertility. We have mentioned infection in relation to the cervical mucus and equally any infection of the vagina must be cleared. It is true to say that such an infection may not provide an absolute bar to conception but nevertheless it may contribute to delay and should be treated.

Sexual counselling may be necessary for some couples and indeed where serious problems exist, for example, impotence, psychiatric help may be required. For a surprising number of couples simple facts on the way things function, when conception is likely to occur, the timing and frequency of intercourse, and so on, are very necessary.

So we can see that many approaches can be made to the problem of female infertility depending on where the problem lies. Careful assessment first of all is a 'must' if successful therapeutic measures are to be applied. If it is found to be a fault in the ovary without regular ovulation occurring then modern day therapy can be applied to stimulate the ovaries into activity. The success of these drugs can be assessed by monitoring methods using either ultrasound scanning or sophisticated laboratory hormone measurements.

If the problem is one of tubal blockage then surgical procedures refined by the use of microscopy may be applied or, more recently and more excitingly, in vitro fertilisation may be used.

Then there are miscellaneous problems leading to or associated with infertility. Fibroids, endometriosis, infection, poor or hostile cervical mucus – all can be identified and corrective measures taken.

It still leaves a group of infertile couples who have to be labelled '*cause unknown*'. This group dwindles in number as expertise in investigation increases. Hopefully it will continue to dwindle. The use of IVF for this group has its advocates and they may be right.

Two aspects of infertility work remain to be mentioned in any discussion on treatment. First, there is *adoption*. Many couples will turn to adoption agencies in their search for a child. Latest figures show that with changing moral and social attitudes and with the wider use of contraception and abortion fewer than 1000 babies are adopted each year in Britain. Older children and handicapped children are easily available and fortunately many couples will adopt these children in their determination to complete a family unit.

It is possible, of course, that the pendulum may swing back and as IVF and its related procedures become more readily available and more successful, there will be fewer applicants to adopt and those who do will be more quickly provided for.

Then there is *surrogate motherhood*. This means that someone who is capable of pregnancy is fertilised (with the husband's sperm) on behalf of the potential mother, who is infertile, and carries her pregnancy for her. This approach to infertility treatment received official examination in recent times when the Warnock Committee examined and commented on various aspects of infertility work including IVF and all its implications, and surrogacy. The latter is a difficult moral and ethical issue which does not really require amplification so obvious are the problems. Suffice it to say that as an official, legal and ethically acceptable method of therapy in infertility work it is, as yet, a non-starter.

# 8

# Related Problems

There are several clinical problems which are related to, and indeed may be presented to the doctor as, infertility. We have already looked at *pelvic inflammatory disease* (p. 36), so common in modern permissive times. Here the end result is, at worst, blockage of the tubes and, at least, adhesions limiting the motility and function of the tubes. Surgery may or may not be possible but IVF provides an increasingly attractive and successful option in the management of infertility due to this distressing condition.

We have also looked at the curious phenomenon of *endometriosis* (p. 36) where patches of endometrial cells grow outside the uterine cavity, usually in the pelvis, on the ovary and surrounding the base of the uterus. Adhesions may result, cysts of the ovary may develop and in any case, although patency of the tubes may remain, absolute or relative infertility can be associated with the condition. Modern drugs, especially danazol, can transform the outcome of this disease so far as fertility is concerned.

There remain two important problems to consider. First, the problem of *recurrent abortion* and, second, the problem of *amenorrhoea*.

**Recurrent abortion**

Sometimes called habitual abortion this means three or more spontaneous abortions and requires investigation. The abortions must take place before 28 weeks, of course.

Spontaneous abortion is, in fact, the most common complication of pregnancy. Of all recognisable pregnancies 15 per cent end within the first three months, although the rate is probably much higher since many pregnancies and abortions will go unrecognised. It has been estimated that the frequency of recurrent abortion is somewhere in the region of 0.4 to 0.8 per cent. What are the recognised reasons for recurrent abortions – 'recognised' because in many couples no cause will be identified?

### CAUSES OF RECURRENT ABORTION

*Genetic*

Abnormalities in chromosome structure or numbers accounts for over 50 per cent of early abortions. Nowadays if such an abnormality is detected in the products of an early abortion a similar abnormality should be excluded if possible in a subsequent pregnancy – by chorionic villus sampling for example. An examination of the woman's chromosomes – and her partner's – will be a test that is carried out.

*Anatomical*

*Abnormalities of development* of the fetus tend to lead to abortion. Severe developmental abnormalities almost always do so though less severe anormalities such as spina bifida may not. Fortunately the detection of such abnormalities is nowadays made possible by blood tests on the mother (alphafetoprotein measurement) or by careful ultrasound scanning.

Abnormalities of maternal anatomy may be incriminated. Perhaps the best known one is *cervical incompetence*. This means what it says – the cervix, the neck of the womb, is incompetent to hold in a pregnancy and the typical story is that the pregnancy 'drops out' (often almost literally) usually in the second trimester, after 12 weeks of pregnancy.

A typical background history to such a situation is that there has been some form of surgery to the cervix some time previously. A common procedure is dilatation and curettage and sometimes the dilatation part of the operation over-dilates the cervix so that it never returns to its former competent state.

Fortunately this situation is treatable and a 'purse-string' stitch, called a Shirodkar suture after its Indian inventor, can be inserted round the base of the cervix and tied firmly. This hopefully holds in the pregnancy until two weeks before term, when the stitch is removed.

*Abnormalities of uterine development* may rarely be a reason for recurrent abortion. The development of the uterus is in two halves which fuse together with, ultimately, breakdown of the fused walls so as to form a single cavity. If this breakdown does not occur then there may be left a two-chambered uterus – a bicornuate uterus – or the cavity may have a complete or partial septum dividing it (see Fig. 5/3, p. 56).

These kinds of developmental abnormalities, however, do not by any means all result in abortions. Certainly in a patient with recurrent abortions, an abnormal uterus such as we have described, and no other detectable abnormalities, then careful consideration will be given to surgical repair. But not at all infrequently women with such abnormalities carry their pregnancies successfully to term.

Other abnormalities of the cavity of the uterus may be produced by fibroids which can distort the cavity. Once again it must be said that not all fibroids will lead to abortion.

The operation to remove fibroids – myomectomy – will be reserved for women when no other problems can be detected and where the fibroids are growing under the lining of the womb and therefore distort the shape of the cavity.

### *Infections*

It is doubtful just how much part maternal infections of the genital tract play in recurrent abortion. Nevertheless many authorities would say that it is important to exclude any infection of the lining of the womb – an *endometritis*.

*Blood incompatibility*
In a Rhesus negative woman with a Rhesus positive husband there may be a possibility that the baby's blood is Rhesus positive (under certain circumstances which do not concern us here, it may be Rhesus negative). Antibodies to the baby's blood may develop in the mother's blood which can then return into the baby's circulation causing breakdown of its blood. If the mother has extremely high levels of antibodies (built up as a result of previous pregnancies) it is possible for the baby to succumb before 28 weeks.

But this is very rare nowadays. For one thing, modern management of Rhesus negative mothers is such that at any procedure (birth itself, for example) where a shower of the baby's blood cells can be expected to enter the mother's bloodstream, a protective injection (called Anti-D) can be given to the mother to clear her bloodstream of these invading cells and thereby avoid the development of antibodies.

In mothers who have already developed antibodies a watch can be kept on the state of the baby from an early stage in pregnancy and sophisticated methods now allow doctors to 'top up' an affected baby with Rhesus negative blood while it is still in the uterus.

The part which ABO blood group incompatibility plays in recurrent abortion is less certain.

*Endocrine*
The part which progesterone hormone deficiency plays in abortion and recurrent abortion in particular is still debated and there is no clear-cut answer. Nevertheless, some doctors will recommend weekly injections of progesterone and certainly the mother concerned will feel satisfied that everything possible is being tried to sustain the early pregnancy – a considerable psychological boost apart from anything else.

The only risk to the treatment is in continuing it for too long when masculinisation of a female fetus is a possibility.

Other endocrine conditions such as diabetes and thyroid disease need identification and treating in their own right, but in the uncontrolled state these diseases may indeed lead to recurrent abortion.

*Immunological*

The study of the immunology of pregnancy is a relatively new one and of such complexity that any attempt at detailed explanation will not be made here. But one basic question needs to be answered – why does the mother not always reject her pregnancy when, after all, it can be likened to a grafted kidney which will certainly be rejected by the host body if certain immunological steps are not taken?

In successful pregnancies it seems that in some way the mother produces 'blocking' antibodies to the 'immune attack' on the foreign graft that is her pregnancy. It has been suggested that maternal failure to produce such blocking antibody is the problem in many women suffering from recurrent abortions. In a recent, carefully controlled trial women with such a history were immunised with paternal white blood cells and the results have been successful in a significant number of women. Much work remains to be done along these lines but progress is encouraging.

**Amenorrhoea**

Let us look at the problem of amenorrhoea now. Usually but not always, if regular menstruation is not taking place then ovulation is not occurring either.

*Primary amenorrhoea* is where menstruation has never taken place and of course is normal before the menarche. If by 18 years of age no menstruation has occurred then investigations will begin.

*Secondary amenorrhoea* is where menstruation has been

occurring normally and then has been absent for six months or longer.

Both types have some causal factors in common. The possible causes and their investigations and treatment are now outlined underlining, when appropriate, where primary or secondary amenorrhoea is likely to be involved.

### PHYSIOLOGICAL CAUSES (I.E. 'NATURAL')

The most obvious example is pregnancy and this has to be thought of in both primary and secondary amenorrhoea although it is obviously much more common in the latter.

Investigation: Standard pregnancy tests
Ultrasound

### ABNORMALITIES OF UTERUS OR VAGINA

The best-known example here is the so-called 'imperforate hymen' where a thin membrane obstructs the outlet of the vagina.

Investigation: History
Examination: under anaesthesia if necessary

Treatment: Excise the membrane

A rare cause is absence of a vagina. Treatment is to create a functional vagina surgically.

An 'obstructive' cause which we have already mentioned in another context is Asherman's syndrome where the cavity of the uterus is occluded by adhesions.

Treatment: Breakdown of adhesions surgically, *or* by insertion of an intrauterine contraceptive device

### ABNORMALITIES OF THE OVARY

Chromosome abnormalities involving ovarian function will largely give rise to primary amenorrhoea. There is no treatment.

Unfortunately a premature menopause – even in quite young women – may be a cause of secondary amenorrhoea. There is no treatment, but undesirable symptoms such as hot flushes can be treated with hormone replacement therapy.

PITUITARY GLAND DISORDERS

Tumours (often 'micro' tumours) of the pituitary may cause a rise in the level of the hormone called prolactin and this in turn produces amenorrhoea – usually secondary.

| | |
|---|---|
| Investigation: | Skull *x*-rays |
| Treatment: | The drug bromocriptine reduces the level of prolactin, menstruation and ovulation usually follow<br>Larger tumours need to be removed surgically or by radiotherapy |

Other gland problems may result in amenorrhoea. Notable in this respect is a poorly-acting thyroid gland – hypothyroidism.

| | |
|---|---|
| Investigation: | Measure the activity of the thyroid by blood tests |
| Treatment: | Give thyroid extract |

DISORDERS OF THE HYPOTHALAMUS

'Stress' is arguably the most common reason at present for amenorrhoea. This includes stress of all kinds – family problems, personal upsets, work worries, new jobs, first jobs and so on. Typically, nurses just starting on their hard and demanding work experience a time of amenorrhoea, and students finishing their studies and starting work in a new and unfamiliar environment.

One of the best known problems leading to amenorrhoea is anorexia nervosa where, typically, young women become almost obsessed by their body image and voluntarily starve themselves in order to lose weight. Amenorrhoea almost always results. Equally in girls who 'crash diet' from time to time a period of amenorrhoea may follow.

It has to be remembered, however, that at the other end of the scale overweight may cause if not outright amenorrhoea then certainly oligomenorrhoea which means scanty irregular periods. This has the same end result of lack of ovulation and failure to conceive.

Amenorrhoea may follow cessation of the contraceptive pill for a time – for a reason that is not entirely clear. Naturally this is distressing for those women who may have come off the pill for the purpose of becoming pregnant. Fortunately

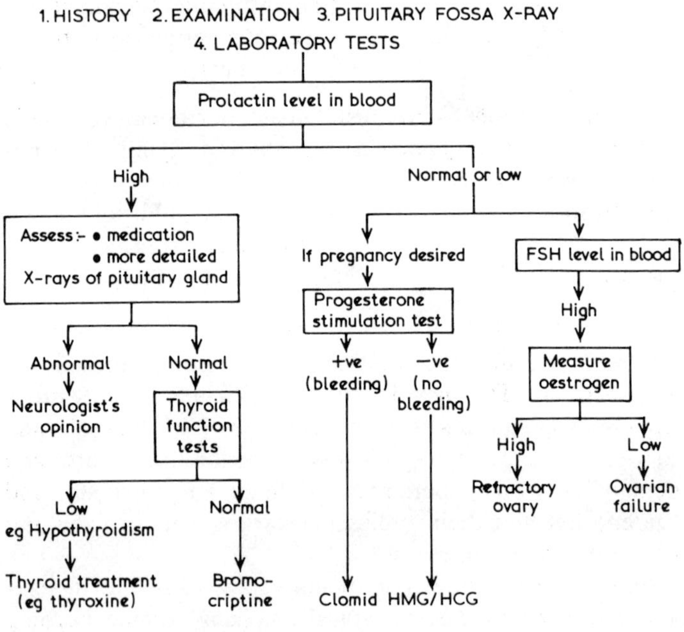


Table 8/1 Investigations and treatment of amenorrhoea

if it does not correct itself it is easily treatable with the drug Clomid.

Table 8/1 shows the pattern of investigation for a woman who stops having her periods and these investigations will be followed particularly in the woman who desires to start a pregnancy. It also shows the available treatment for such women especially if pregnancy is the desired outcome for such investigations.

# 9

# The Future

And what of future progress in the successful management of problems of infertility? We need look only at the advances of the recent past to see that we are in the midst of progress now, and very exciting it is.

Recent advances lie in several fields. First of all our knowledge of what can go wrong has been advanced by the development of more sophisticated techniques in the laboratory.

Measurements of hormones have been developed and are now commonly available. Laboratory techniques too have clarified our knowledge of the glandular hormonal control of conception and of the influence of other intrinsic or external factors on that control.

A recent development has been in the use of ultrasound scanning to follow the functioning of the ovary and to scrutinise the pelvic organs and their state of normality or otherwise. The laparoscope, by which we can clearly see the state of the pelvic organs and examine, in particular, the tubes and their appearance and test their patency, has been an advance of the last dozen years or so.

Surgical techniques for the repair of damaged tubes in particular has been advancing rapidly since the development of microsurgical techniques. Overtaking it, however, is the latest and most exciting advance of all – in vitro fertilisation. With all its drawbacks, the philosophical and ethical doubts which accompany it, this technique must surely be the greatest single hope for women whose apparent infertility is based on damaged tubes.

The testing of immunological theories especially in the realm of recurrent abortion problems is at present proving exciting, as we have seen.

It is difficult to be a forecaster of the future in things medical and in the context of infertility this is particularly true. Other commentators will undoubtedly draw attention to other areas of likely progress but the writer would like to make the following – hopefully encouraging – prognostications for the future.

First, in male infertility much remains to be done. Further progress in the control of and therefore the improvement of spermatogenesis is likely to develop. Hormone involvement in these factors remains to be elucidated in certain areas so that there is greater availability of treatment. Increasing interest in and understanding of male sexual problems is already advancing rapidly and a much more active line taken in management.

Then continuing study of the function of the ovary will, it is certain, lead to valuable progress in treatment of ovulation failure. Is ovulation always 'adequate'? This is a situation that is already recognised – and more needs to be learned about it.

The drugs at present used to stimulate ovulation – Clomid, HMG and HCG – are good but the last is not without its problems. Further development in this direction should lead to safer, easier to use and more effective 'fertility drugs'. The easier identification of ovulation needs to be devised and indeed a prediction test for the potential mother to use so that intercourse can occur (with optimism!) at the correct timing, is an advance which is likely to be achieved in the near future.

The most immediate advances are likely to be made in the field of in vitro fertilisation. The technique of harvesting the eggs, of the laboratory methods of fertilisation, of reimplantation – how and where – and so on, will go on improving. Most importantly of all it is to be hoped that these facilities and the availability of these skills will become much more widespread among our community. In such a worthwhile area of medical therapy where great strain and sadness among couples can potentially be relieved it seems unthinkable that adequate funds will not be made available for such progressive work.

# Suggested Further Reading

Llewellyn-Jones, D. (1982). *Every Man*. Oxford University Press, Oxford.

Llewellyn-Jones, D. (1986). *Everywoman*, 4th edition. Faber and Faber, London.

# Index